HOW TO SLOW DOWN CELL AGING

And Live Healthier For Longer

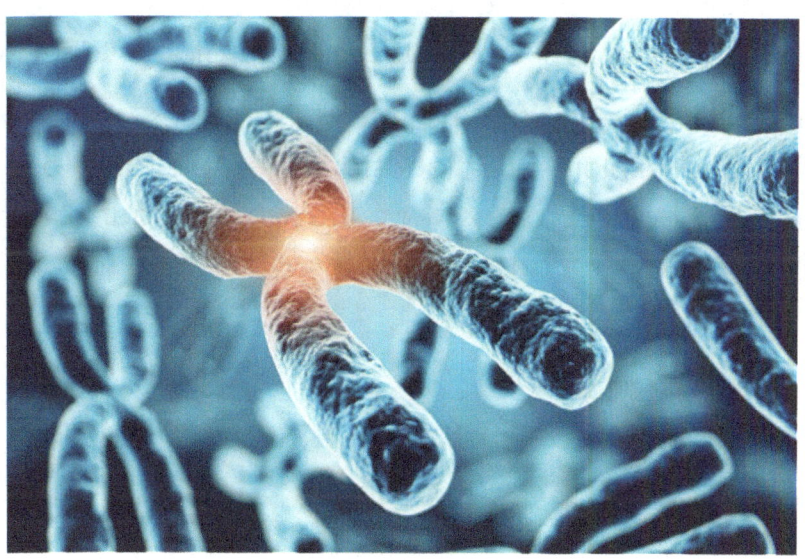

What really works according to science?

Aging doesn't have to be something we just accept. Research shows it might actually be a treatable "disease."

In this book, we'll share the latest discoveries about anti-aging and explore practical steps we can take to slow down the aging process while we wait for that ultimate genetic breakthrough.

TABLE OF CONTENTS

INTRODUCTION 1
WHY DO WE AGE? 2
LIFESTYLE 5
NUTRITION 13
SUPPLEMENTS 23
SUPPLEMENTATION PROGRAMS 82
EPIGENETIC DIET 86
TYPICALLY ANTIOXIDANT FOODS 102
COSMETICS 104
CONCLUSIONS 110
DISCLAIMER 111
REFERENCES 112

INTRODUCTION

Modern science has certainly helped us live longer, but let's be clear: we're really just *extending old age*, which is a different story altogether. While we may add years to our lives, those later years aren't always spent in great health.

Most of us don't start worrying about our old age until we hit 50, and here's the kicker: conventional medicine often looks at our lifestyles and health predictions only for the next few years.

We are unaware of it, but already after the age of twenty, our arteries begin to degrade, most likely without any harmful consequences before reaching the age of sixty. Still, if we immediately start to take care of the proper functioning of our organism, we can delay (and for a long time) the appearance of those disorders that are the leading cause of natural death. Therefore, we obtain double the result of living longer and having better health.

So, when is the best time to start worrying about the consequences for our health in old age? The answer is: "*The best time was yesterday.*"

We start shaping our health from childhood, so the sooner we start paying attention to it, the better off we'll be later.

Above all, it is important to take a **holistic** approach that covers everything: good nutrition, healthy lifestyles, adequate exercise, a personalized integration program, attention to the emotional-psychological sphere, and basic skincare.

WHY DO WE AGE?

Every single eukaryotic (Contributors to Wikimedia projects, 2001) cell in our body has a nucleus. Inside this nucleus, you'll find chromosomes packed with genetic information—our DNA. When the cell replicates, it copies all that information, but there's an exception: the end of the chromosomes, known as **telomeres**.

Telomeres protect the end of chromosomes and prevent the DNA helix from flaking at any cellular duplication. Without telomeres, essential information about the genetic code would be lost when the cell replicates.

At the two ends of the DNA double helix, we, therefore, find telomeres, which do not carry information (such as how to produce proteins of genetic interest, etc.) but protect the rest of the strand from disintegration, like "caps" they, therefore, preserve our chromosomes.

The problem is that at each cell replication, these telomeres are consumed, shortening each time until reaching a critical threshold beyond which the cell can no longer divide; therefore, it is destined to die (in some cases, instead of dying, it continues to wander in our body as a senescent cell causing dangerous damage to our health).

When it dies, we lose not just its specific function but the block of information it carries. This means our body struggles to create new cells, which is one of the reasons why we start to "age."

Science has recently discovered that there is a potential to slow telomere shortening. This is done naturally in our body by an enzyme called **telomerase**. It has been discovered that this enzyme is present in all our cells, but in most of our tissues, it is not very active, while it is most active in the germ cells (therefore ova and spermatozoa) and stem cells.

In these specific cells, the telomeres undergo a much smaller shortening than the rest of our body.

The question is:

Is there the possibility of activating telomerase in other cells as well?

There's a lot of exciting research on telomerase now. Many scientists have conducted a lot of experiments (both in vitro and on mice), and the discoveries made so far are promising. Researchers believe we'll be able to control telomerase within the next ten years.

However, there are still many issues to solve before finding a way to intervene directly in the genetic code. Still, along the research path, several ways have been identified to at least slow down the telomere shortening process and enhance telomerase in our cells, thus allowing us to obtain a real slowdown in the aging process of our body.

Another important cause of aging is that, slowly but surely, the cells, over time, take on a characteristic secretory phenotype (SASP), which feeds the chronic pro-inflammatory state of the whole organism.

This chronic systemic inflammation compromises the regenerative capacity of stem cells and consequently increases the risk of developing various age-related diseases.

In fact, with aging, senescent cells accumulate in many tissues and pathology sites of many chronic diseases.

Therefore, current anti-aging research is strongly oriented toward discovering and using molecules capable of eliminating senescent cells or at least reducing their secretory phenotype (anti-SASP).

While waiting for scientific research to provide us with the keys to a controlled genetic modification, there are currently different several ways to limit the damage of cellular aging by acting on **inflammation** (which has devastating effects on our body), **oxidation**, **immune system**, and **insulin sensitivity**.

This can be achieved by intervening in three fields:

- Lifestyle
- Diet
- Supplements

LIFESTYLE

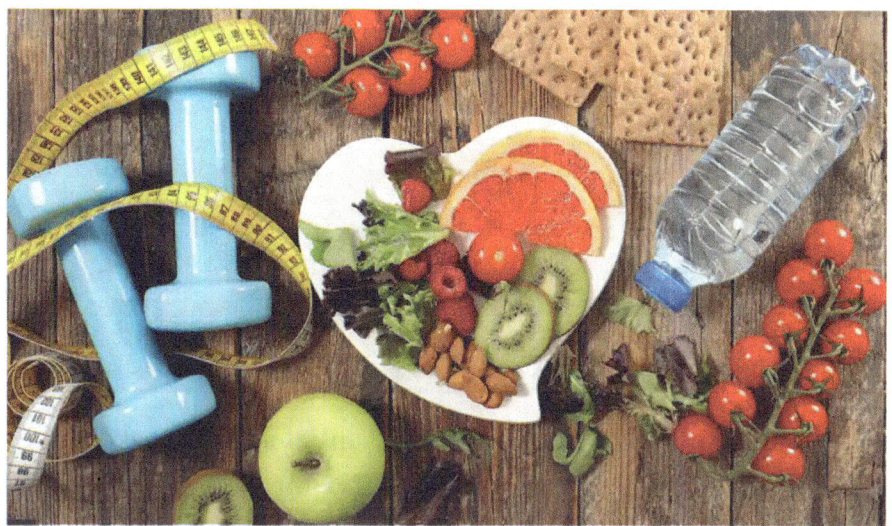

Our lifestyle can profoundly affect our cells' aging rate both in the negative and positive sense.

Given that, obviously, we are all different. The biological clock of each of us moves at different speeds (and the responses of our bodies to the same solicitations can be very different from one person to another); this does not detract from the fact that in the range of our genetic possibilities, you can do a lot for your health and your biological age (a lot of good or a lot of bad ...).

Let's start with the **negative factors**.

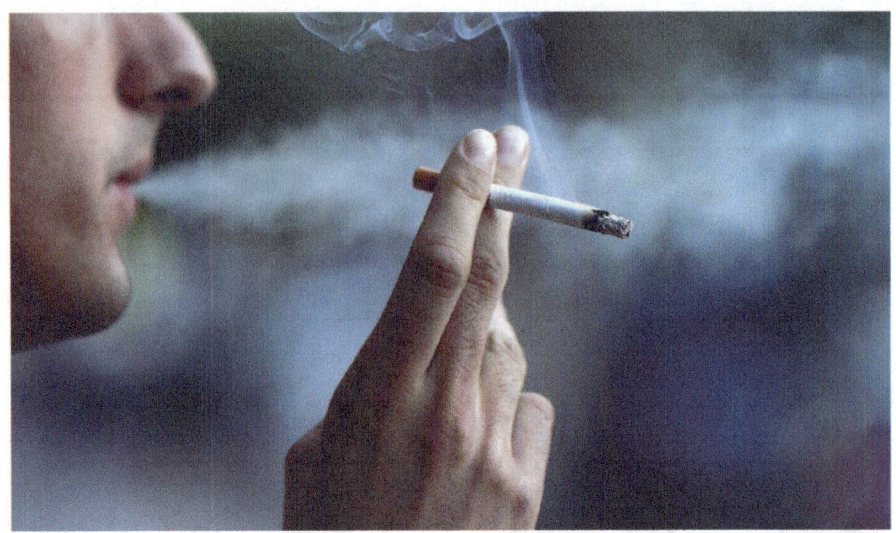

First of all, **smoking**. Smoking speeds up telomeres breakdown by three to five times that of non-smokers. In addition to inducing addiction, nicotine also has harmful effects on the cardiovascular system because it causes damage to the blood vessels, causing arterial hypertension, stroke, ischemic heart disease, heart failure, and aortic aneurysm. Not to mention the effects of skin aging.

Quitting smoking should, therefore, be the first step in a solid anti-aging program.

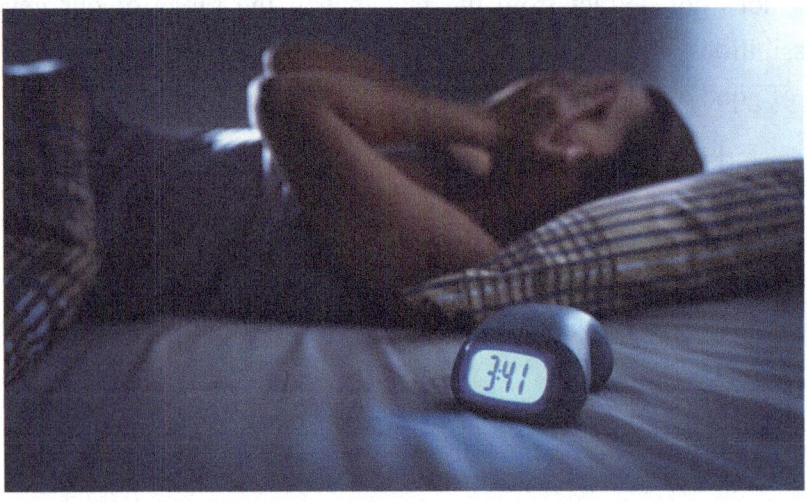

The second harmful practice is **poor sleep**. It has been seen that in those who sleep less than six hours a night, there is a sharp shortening of the telomeres, especially of a particular type of lymphocyte (a cell of our immune system), which, when it gets older, exposes us to both bacterial and viral infections.

Extensive studies have shown that lack of sleep promotes cardiovascular and cognitive pathologies, as well as has negative effects on insulin sensitivity.

Among other things, sleeping little also has catabolic (disintegration) effects on our muscle tissue.

We should sleep at least seven to eight hours a night to get the maximum positive effect (better to sleep on the side: preferring and maintaining the habit of sleeping on the left side would have positive consequences on both health and longevity resting by placing the left side on the mattress would generally improve lymphatic drainage, digestion, and circulation).

In general, women need about 20-30 minutes more sleep on average than men. So if you want to improve the quality of sleep, consider trying *yoga nidra* and meditation. Later, we'll check out some supplements that can help you sleep better.

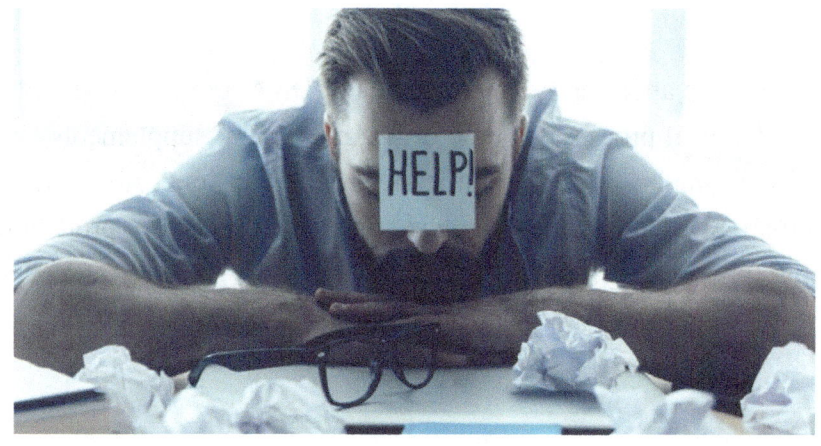

The third element that speeds up telomeres shortening is **chronic stress**.

It has been widely demonstrated that living in a situation of prolonged chronic stress, significantly increases the production of cortisol (Contributors to Wikimedia projects, 2003), which in turn has largely destructive effects on our bodies.

Therefore, managing stress and emotional state is essential to slow down aging.

Practices of diaphragmatic breathing (Johnson, 2020), digital pressure, and meditation are beneficial for this purpose. Numerous studies have shown that practicing meditation, even for just 15 minutes daily, increases telomerase activity.

It could be argued that many people have no control over their quality of life and, consequently, their stress. This is true, but daily observation shows us that there are people who would not have particular reasons to be stressed, and yet they are at extreme levels, as well as there are individuals who, on the contrary, would have all the reasons but are much less stressed than most people.

Science has amply demonstrated that what we call "stress," even before being of psychological origin, is a genetic and chemical-biological issue.

We cannot do anything (yet) to change our DNA, but we can intervene in biochemical processes. Some drugs and natural supplements (such as Ashwagandha) have significant effects on our stress levels. Alternatively, we can take supplements that limit cortisol production, such as phosphatidylserine.

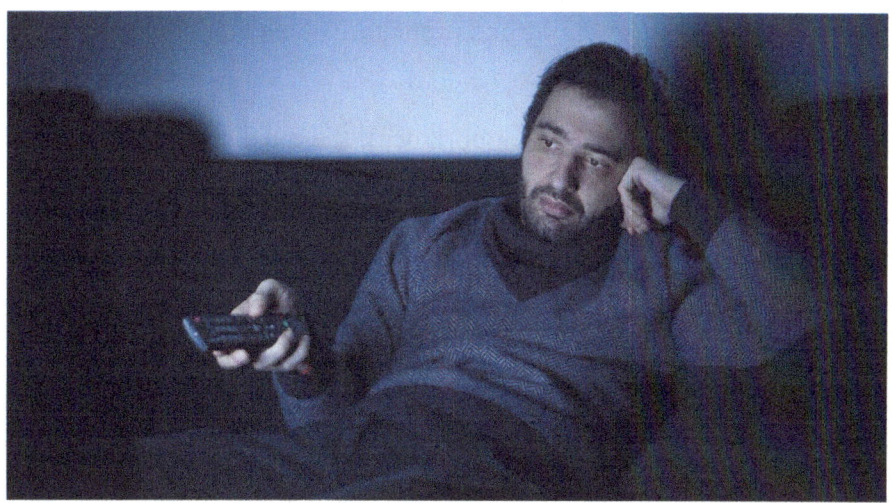

Little **physical activity** (or absence) also causes the telomeres to be shorter.

Numerous studies have shown that those who practice sports even for only 30 minutes three times a week, compared to those who do not, are found to have telomeres significantly longer.

What type of activity to choose? Long-standing is the rant: better cardio or weights? Recent studies published in the *British Journal of Sports Medicine* have shown that the best anti-aging results are obtained with a **combination of the two**.

In both cases, the activity should not be too intense, as the free radicals produced by excessive effort would nullify the benefits of exercise.

Yoga is strongly recommended as it also has a powerful anti-stress effect.

Among other things, doing a pleasant physical activity reduces stress (*any pleasant physical activity*) and improves insulin sensitivity (ScienceDirect, n.d.).

The risk of death for those who do not exercise is approximately 200% higher than those who exercise regularly. In practice, the absence of physical activity causes aging and premature death more than any other incorrect behavior.

Specifically (and in order of importance), the most significant factors are VO2 Max (VO2 Max Testing Exercise Physiology Core Laboratory, n.d.) (the maximum volume of oxygen that a person can consume per unit of time per muscle contraction), strength, and muscle mass.

VO2 Max

Several studies suggest that the most useful way to improve VO2 Max is HIIT (High Intensity Interval Training) (Contributors to Wikimedia projects, 2005). This is because HIIT forces us to temporarily reach or exceed the anaerobic threshold before returning to a lower, aerobic intensity. This type of overload causes the heart and lungs to quickly adapt to the stress they are subjected to. The direct consequence is that VO2 Max increases.

Strength

Strength is achieved by reaching high levels of muscular tension. Typically, a training session is done with many sets of few repetitions with a weight very close to your maximum (80% 90%), for example, 5/6 sets of 3/5 repetitions.

Muscle mass

The maximum stimulus for muscle hypertrophy is obtained with a workout of about 3 sets of 8/10 repetitions, using weights at 70-75% of your maximum.

The amount of protein consumed daily is fundamental for muscle growth (recent studies have shown that the older you get, the more the demand for proteins increases as we become metabolically resistant to protein synthesis).

Extremely useful for muscle hypertrophy is the integration of good doses of creatine (3 to 5 g per day). Creatine has also proven to be very interesting from an anti-aging point of view, as recent studies have shown that it has anti-inflammatory and anti-catabolic action.

Other useful tips:

- **Walking barefoot on the bare ground:** This produces numerous benefits both in terms of magnetism and the alkaline balance of our organism. We recommend walking with a long stride, not necessarily fast but wide (it is noticeable how, as people get older, their stride becomes shorter and shorter, so try to keep a long stride to keep your muscles and sense of balance effective).
- **Deep breathing:** On an empty stomach, lying face up or sitting, eyes closed, take deep breaths starting with diaphragmatic breathing (therefore filling the stomach with air) through the nose, continuing by filling the lungs (maximum opening of the chest), and finally bringing the air in the head. Hold your breath for a few seconds (according to our possibilities) and exhale vigorously through your mouth, reopening your eyes. Hold for a few seconds with empty lungs and start again.
- **Sun exposure at dawn and dusk:** Advantages: low levels of UV, endogenous production of vitamin D3, lower cortisol levels, maximum levels of red light (which is anti-inflammatory and stimulates the production of collagen and elastin).
- **Train preferably in the morning**; acceptable in the afternoon; absolutely not in the evening (doing sports in the evening has negative effects, among other things, on the quality of sleep).

- **Positive lifestyles** are about making healthier choices, which is clearly the opposite of what has been stated before. So, quit smoking, sleep regularly—at least 7/8 hours a night— and find a way to reduce stress. Don't forget to get moving with regular physical activity.

On top of that, try to get some sunlight, breathe (as much as possible) fresh, good-quality air, and cultivate social relationships and hobbies that bring us satisfaction and pleasure.

Social relationships are essential to living healthily for a long time. It results from a new study published in the "Proceedings of the National Academy of Sciences." From an extensive analysis of thousands of subjects, followed for many years, it has clearly emerged that the quantity and quality of social relationships are positively correlated with good health and longevity.

If possible, try to hang out with people younger than you.

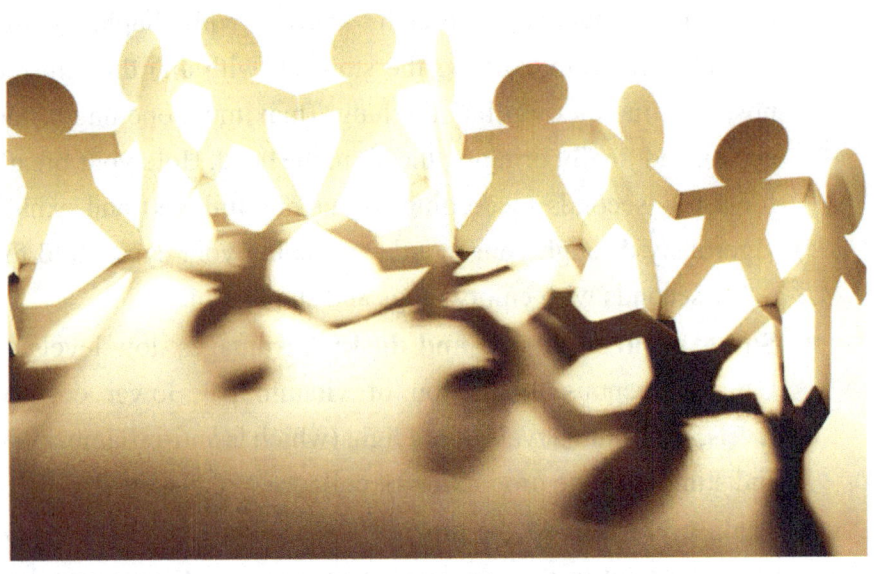

NUTRITION

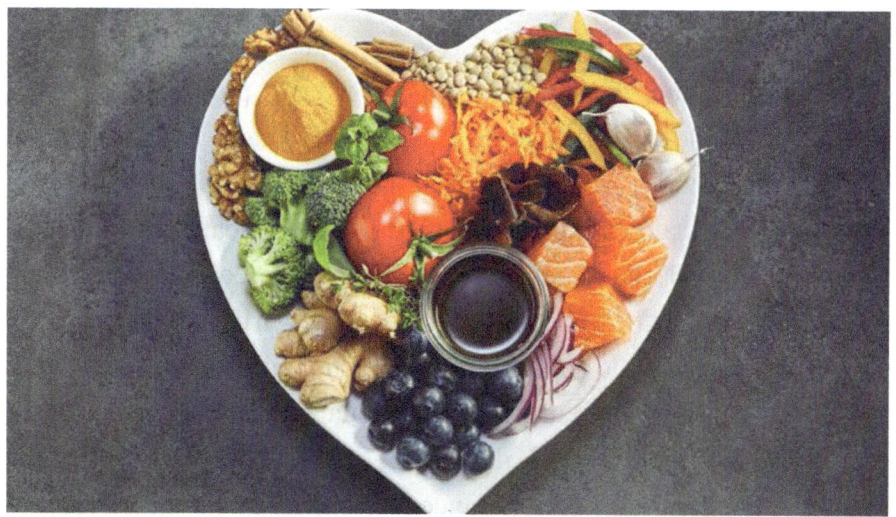

An incorrect diet dramatically speeds up the shortening of telomeres, particularly a pro-inflammatory diet, which is, therefore, rich in sugars, processed industrial foods, and trans fats.

The presence of visceral fat also has adverse effects on our telomeres. Visceral fat is the fat we accumulate in the abdomen; it is a subtly more dangerous fat than the fat we accumulate in the rest of the body, as visceral fat is linked to insulin sensitivity. In fact, it has been seen that people with diabetes have shorter telomeres than non-diabetics. Therefore, **improving insulin sensitivity is essential** in order to slow down cellular aging.

In our book "The Whole Truth About Weight Loss," you will find numerous tips on how to improve insulin sensitivity.

We must, therefore, follow a correct diet to slow down aging. By *correct diet,* we mean a diet rich in antioxidants, polyphenols, and

Omega 3 (therefore, legumes, fish, seeds, and fruit) and drinking lots of water (possibly not from plastic bottles).

What to eat:

- reduce the consumption of meat and prefer proteins of vegetable origin (legumes) and milk (better goat's milk) and eggs choose vegetables rich in polyphenols (they activate sirtuins) such as spinach, arugula, broccoli, cabbage, tomatoes eat "good" fats such as olive oil, nuts, seeds in general and Greek yogurt drink green tea consume garlic regularly (garlic contains caffeic acid: caffeic acid is not only an antioxidant but also anti-inflammatory and anti-mutagenic, which means it can reduce the risk of developing cancer. According to the American Institute for Cancer Research, compounds found in garlic can reduce inflammation and contribute to DNA repair, two critical factors in cancer prevention. Garlic is also rich in phytochemicals, including allicin, which can prevent the uncontrolled proliferation of cells and fight fungi and bacteria resistant to antibiotics. What we have seen is that chopping or crushing garlic is essential to obtain the maximum benefits of this substance, so the next time a recipe calls for a clove of garlic, the best thing is to chop or mince it and then keep it away from heat before adding it to the recipe – there are also garlic supplements for those who do not want to have bad breath problems)
- parsley and rosemary (see dedicated chapters later)
- salmon and avocado (see dedicated chapters later)

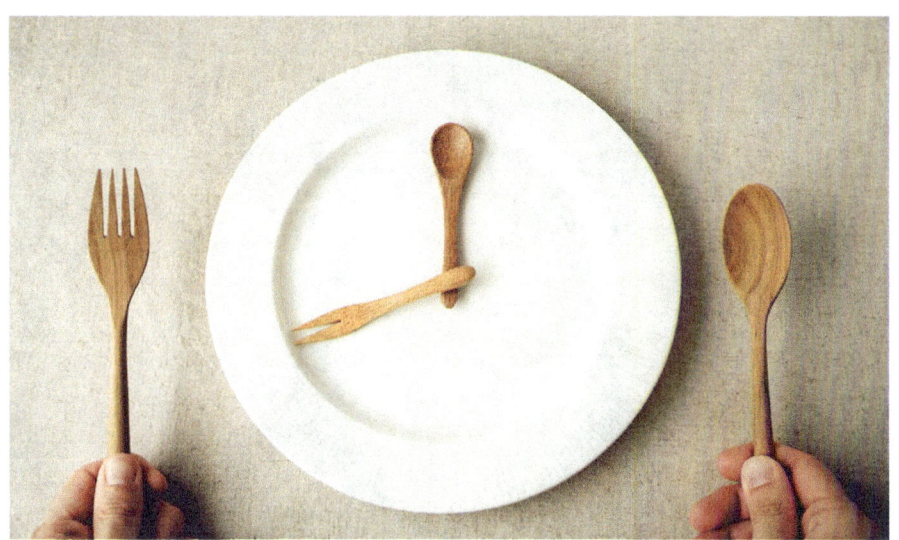

Intermittent fasting can also be helpful for our purposes. In fact, it has been seen that short fasts of even only 12-16 hours allow an increase in the production of stem cells, and, as we said previously, stem cells are among the few in our body that have telomerase always active, therefore increasing the stem cells extend the life of our organism.

Furthermore, during fasting, the body produces the GH hormone, a hormone that we usually produce at maximum levels in our 20s but which then decreases drastically as the years go by. Also, the body cleans itself of toxins and inflammation due to overeating. It is essential to drink plenty of water (possibly not cold) during fasting.

Ideally, two meals a day, mid-morning and mid-afternoon (according to some studies, it would be advisable not to eat after sunset).

NB: Your body will need at least a couple of weeks to adapt to this new nutritional cycle.

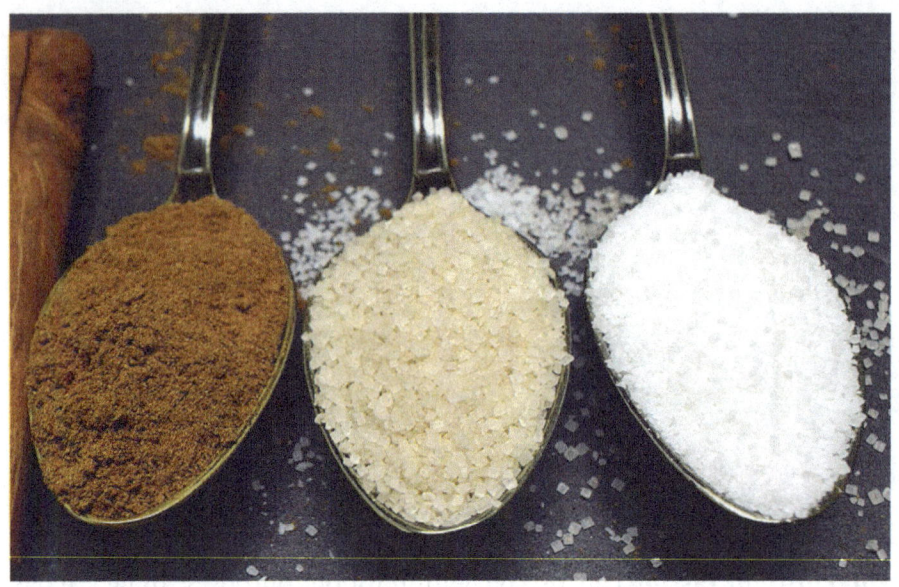

Sugar deserves a separate chapter.

Sugar is a real poison for our health that we must literally banish from our tables. Let's see why.

Immediate effects:

The intake of even a modest amount of sugar causes a sudden rise in blood sugar in our body, which reacts with an equally rapid overproduction of insulin.

Medium-term effects and increased risk of developing diseases:

If repeated over time on a continuous basis, this phenomenon is not well tolerated: the mechanism tends to become saturated, leading to a greater risk of developing insulin resistance or a lower efficacy of insulin. Overweight, obesity, and the general inflammatory state of the body are interrelated.

Long-term effects and chronic diseases:

The development of chronic diseases such as diabetes leads to metabolic syndrome and certain types of cancer.

There are also many other harmful side effects of excessive sugar intake, such as damage to the skin. In fact, the excess sugar makes it easier to bond with the body proteins, resulting in the structural alteration and loss of functionality of the latter. This process is called *glycation*, and a straightforward example of it is what happens on many people's skin: sugar binds, in particular, to collagen and elastin, two proteins contained in the skin tissue, causing accelerated aging.

Skin aging is a visible manifestation of sugar damage, but what happens to collagen and elastin also occurs in all other tissues of our body.

Brain

Sugars are responsible for the premature aging of this organ. Too much sugar also damages memory: Australian researchers at the University of South Wales Medical Science in Sydney have confirmed that constant sugar consumption can cause permanent brain damage.

Hunger

The consumption of sugars is associated with an increase in appetite. The wrong glycemic balance, that is, the sudden increase in the blood sugar content, determines a series of metabolic responses aimed at increasing the feeling of hunger.

Weight

The increase in body weight is another consequence of the consumption of sugars. In reality, the increase in body weight is associated, beyond the caloric intake, with a change in the body's metabolic balance.

Tooth decay

One of the most painful consequences of consuming sugar is the onset of tooth decay. The bacteria of the oral cavity, in fact, use the sugars introduced with food to multiply and damage our teeth.

Zits

Many dermatological disorders are linked to the consumption of sugars. In part, it is because the bacteria of the skin flora feeding on sugars can proliferate uncontrolled. In part, it is because the hormonal changes induced by excessive sugar consumption could lead to a massive secretion of sebum.

Cystitis

Many infections of the urogenital tract are linked to the continuous consumption of sugars. In these cases, one of the first therapeutic choices is precisely to eliminate sugars from the diet.

Other damages

It can cause a sudden increase in adrenaline, hyperactivity, anxiety, difficulty concentrating, and irritability.

It can significantly increase bad cholesterol at the expense of good cholesterol.

It causes loss of elasticity and tissue function.

It can impair vision.

It makes the skin duller, accentuating wrinkles and dark circles.

It is addictive.

The most recent scientific evidence, to which the WHO also refers, links excessive sugar intake to diseases such as:

- obesity
- high cholesterol
- heart disease
- diabetes

It, therefore, appears to cause the same harm, in terms of deaths and sickness, that smoking and alcohol can cause.

Many people can have bowel problems (as too much sugar can alter the bacterial flora) and suffer from high blood pressure or memory problems. There are also some concerns related to the industrial refining of sugar, a chemical process that could increase cancer risk.

Many people tend to distinguish between white sugar and brown sugar, but there are actually no significant differences.

Constant consumption of sugar inhibits the defense capacity of neutrophils (the white blood cells that function as the body's first line of defense). Also, it decreases the maturation and differentiation of lymphocytes.

Progressive studies have shown that an increased intake of white sugar significantly damages the immune system.

Simple sugars counteract the mineral deposition in the bone by inducing acidosis in the body, which the body counteracts by "breaking down" the calcium carbonate (which has a buffering action) of the bones. This process dramatically weakens the bones, leading to osteoporosis.

Sugars clog the cell's primary metabolism, known as the *Krebs cycle*. This involves the accumulation of sugars in the form of fat, and therefore, obesity, which in men is mainly abdominal, while in women, it occurs more in the thighs and buttocks. The accumulation of fat, especially if abdominal, leads to an increased risk of cardiovascular events, such as heart attack and stroke, the development of breast, colon, and prostate cancer, liver problems such as steatosis, ascites, hypertension, diabetes, and all its complications (blindness, kidney failure, etc.).

In theory, to find sugar in food, it would be enough to read the labels of the products, but often, the difficulty lies in recognizing it: in fact, different names are used to indicate the different types of sugar, but they basically have the same effects on our body. The sugars in the labels can be explicit or shown as additives with abbreviations; here are some: white or dark or cane sugar (sucrose), glucose, fructose, dextrose, maltose, various syrups (glucose-fructose, corn, rice), polyols or sugar alcohols (sorbitol E420, mannitol E421, isomalt E953, maltitol E965, xylitol E967, erythritol E968), acesulfame K (E950), aspartame (E951), cyclamates (E952), saccharin (E954), sucrose.

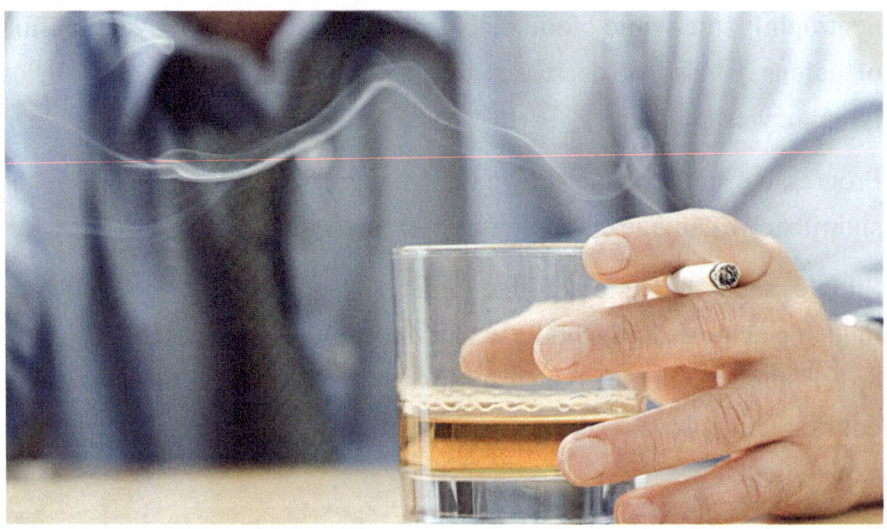

Another food that should be limited (not eliminated but simply *limited)* is **alcohol**.

Chronic excessive alcohol intake, in fact, can have epigenetic effects on our body both at the level of histone (Contributors to Wikimedia projects, 2002) methylation and acetylation, and at the level of micro-RNA modulation.

To give a few examples: according to a 2008 study on humans, alcohol abuse is linked to an over-expression of miR-212. According to other studies, alcohol consumption is linked to an increase in the expression of miR-375 and miR-21 (2009).

These epigenetic changes modify the activity of numerous genes in different brain regions, digestive tract, and liver, which could contribute to developing diseases associated with alcohol abuse and addiction.

Recent studies recommend drinking no more than one glass of wine a day and no more than 4 hours before bedtime (alcohol has devastating consequences on the quality of sleep).

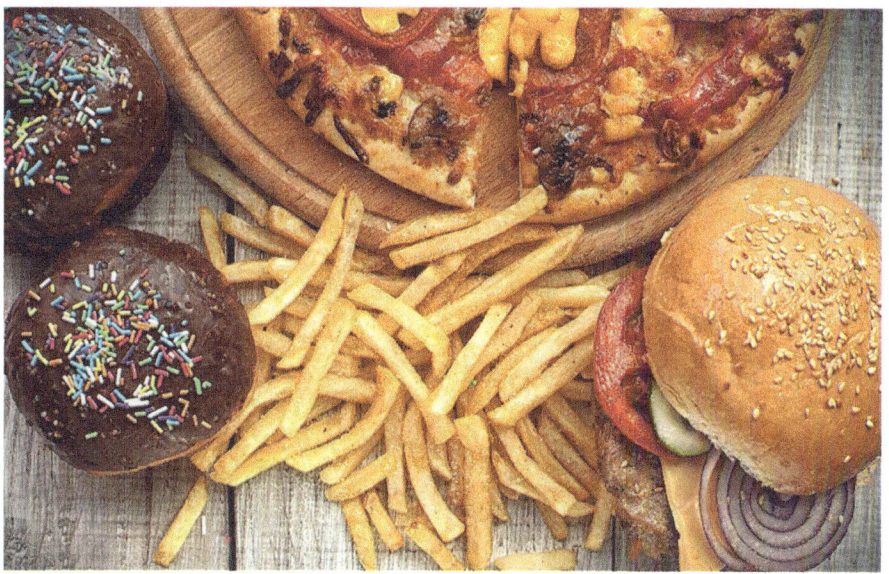

Finally, **saturated fats** should be avoided (or strongly limited): margarine, lard, palm oil, coconut oil, fatty meats (pork belly, sausages), fatty cheeses, fried foods, industrial baked goods (croissants, snacks, sausages, frankfurters, frozen pizza); and instead prefer unsaturated fats (fish, nuts, whole carbohydrates).

Strongly limit bread and pasta with refined flour, cheese, and alcohol (green light for a small quantity of wine every now and then we recommend Pinot Noir, as it is the richest in resveratrol).

Prefer whole fruit (possibly slightly sweet fruit, such as apples and avocado) instead of fruit juices (which generate a strong glycemic spike).

Then, what are the foods that can help us slow down the cellular aging process?

Further on, you will find a chapter dedicated to the *epigenetic diet*.

SUPPLEMENTS

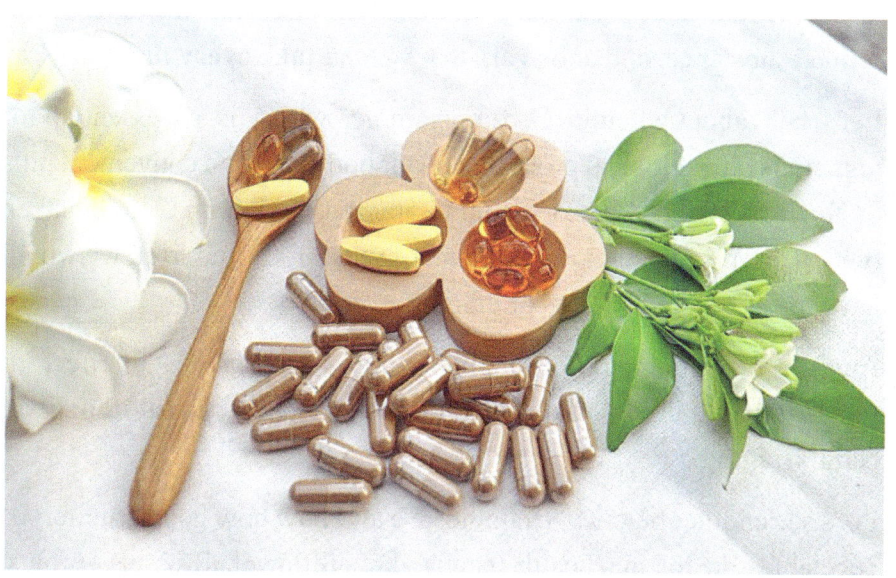

WHY TAKE SUPPLEMENTS?

A timeless myth says that the Mediterranean diet is the best in the world, and that a healthy and varied diet is more than enough to get the vitamins, trace elements, and all the substances we need to stay healthy.

Yes, it undeniably allows you to stay healthy, but does not seriously slow down cellular aging effectively.

Normal nutrition alone cannot provide that boost, that propulsive thrust that would instead be used to slow down our biological clock. We need to give our organism something more.

It is true that if we eat healthily and carefully, we can actually change a lot of the functioning of our organism, but how much can it really change?

The truth is that **diet alone doesn't take you very far**.

We can certainly take vitamins from normal nutrition, but not in the quantities that can be reached with a supplement, with an extracted and refined substance, and above all, that we can **take every day**.

Let's talk about vitamin C, for example, which is so essential for numerous physiological processes in our body. We find convenient pills on the market that can provide up to 500 mg of vitamin C (to be taken twice a day). To get the same amount of vitamin C from fruit, we would have to eat five or six kilos of oranges every day ...

And if a certain amount of vitamin is not reached, it has no effect, or rather, it does, but not what we are looking for, that is **a real impact on cellular aging**.

Let's see another practical example. We all know how good cruciferous vegetables do for our health (cabbage, cauliflower, Brussels sprouts, etc.), but still, to get an impacting effect on the anti-inflammatory and antioxidant processes in our body, we should eat about ten kilos of cabbage a day.

On the market, there are very convenient supplements that, in a single tablet, contain the same amount of active ingredients of crucifers contained in 10 kg of cabbage.

Not to mention that many of the fruits and vegetables we eat are **missing important nutrients**. This is often due to factors like acid rain, land degradation, preservation methods, and how food is handled. Sometimes, they can even be contaminated with harmful substances.

And even if nutrition provides all the nutrients we need, they often face barriers at the cellular level, with a clogged extracellular matrix.

Under normal conditions, this matrix forms a three-dimensional structure, like a sponge that surrounds and protects the individual cells of our body, ensuring the proper supply through the blood of oxygen, nutrients, hormones, neuromodulators, drugs, and adequate removal from the tissues of waste products.

However, the cells may not be in the most suitable conditions to use the nutrients ingested with food, as they are victims of oxidative stress.

Even if correct, **simple nutrition may not be enough** in these cases.

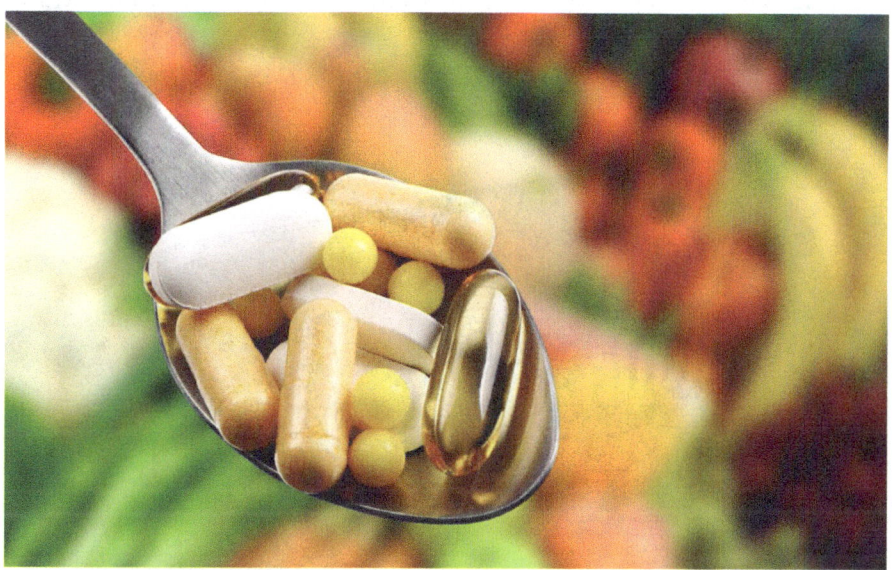

Of course, we will have to take several pills daily, but those pills produce precisely the changes in our bodies that we are looking for: **slowing down cell aging**.

So far, there are no other ways to achieve this, if not in future gene therapy.

Obviously, to work at its best, a **supplement plan must be associated with the lifestyles we discussed in the previous chapter**.

We cannot think of eating french fries with mayonnaise every day, sleeping 5 hours a night, and then expecting to get results just because we are supplementing with vitamins and plant-active ingredients …

WHAT TO TAKE?

Basically, the vitamins that have been shown to be particularly effective are B12, folic acid, vitamin C, vitamin D, vitamin A, and E.

As for trace elements and minerals, magnesium, and zinc have proved helpful because they increase telomerase activity, as well as Omega 3s.

Now, let's look at the substances with **scientifically proven anti-aging capacities** in detail.

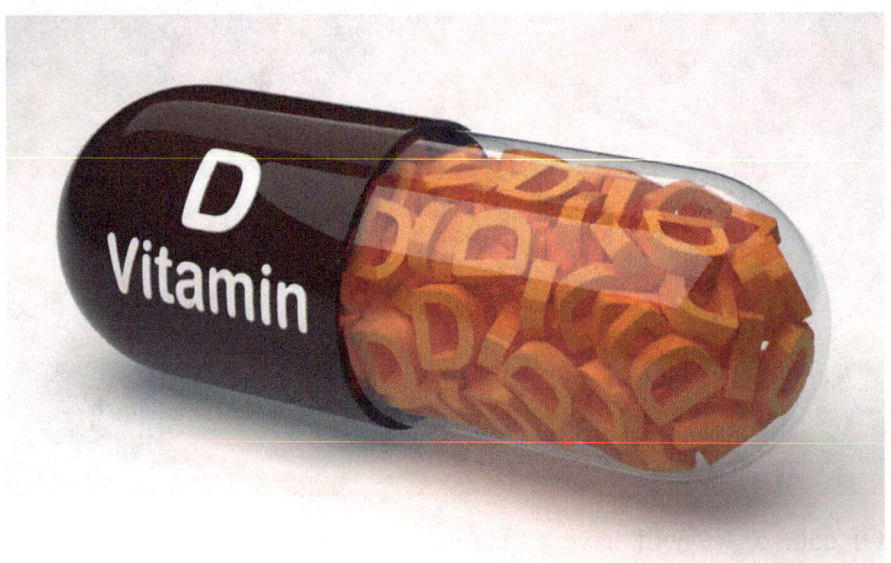

VITAMIN D

Vitamin D isn't just a vitamin; it's actually a pro-hormone. This means it helps control how our genes work. Almost all the cells in our body have vitamin D receptors, which shows how important they are.

One amazing thing about Vitamin D is that it's fat-soluble, so it gets stored in the liver and is released whenever the body needs it—trust me, it's needed in a lot of places! Researchers from Oxford University have found that vitamin D influences over 3,000 different genes, which is really amazing.

We mainly get vitamin D from sunlight; the more skin you expose to the sun and the longer you stay out, the more vitamin D your body makes.

This vitamin is crucial for our immune system, helping us fight off illnesses. It also plays a huge role in reducing intestinal permeability, which can help prevent autoimmune diseases.

Another important function of vitamin D is regulating the amount of calcium available in the body. You can find a lot of vitamin D in the cells of the retina, preserving it from possible damage; in some cases, it was also possible to recover from certain degeneration situations due to the lack of vitamin D itself. Plus, it also has a soothing effect on joint pain.

Why is it necessary to take vitamin D in quantities much higher than what was recommended up to a decade ago?

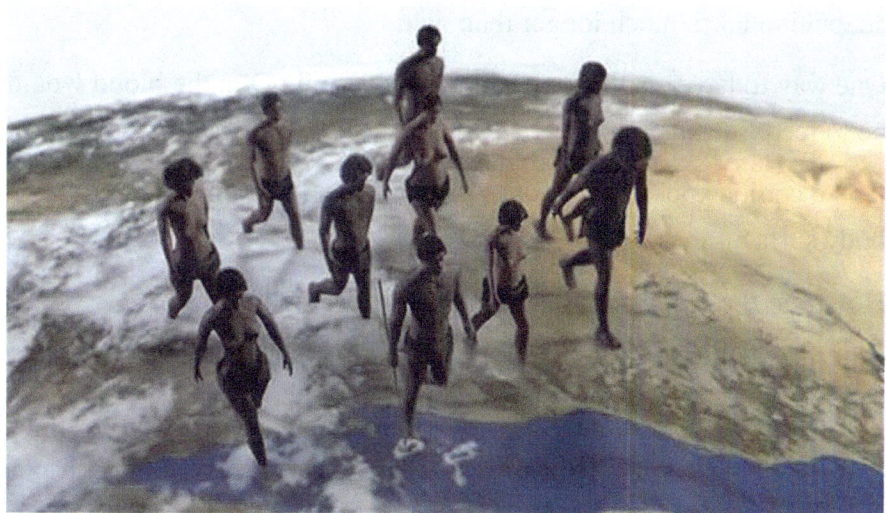

It all started hundreds of thousands of years ago when we were hunter-gatherers in the savannahs of Africa: the sun was much more intense, and we were practically always semi-naked. When we left Africa and moved north to higher latitudes, we had much less sunshine and long, cold winters. At this point, the body, which was used to having a massive amount of vitamin D produced by very intense sun exposure, had to compensate in some way.

The only way was to cut down on the melanin. Thus making the skin progressively clearer and allowing it to absorb more sunlight in less time.

Nevertheless, man has lived for millions of years in conditions typical of the African savannah; therefore, vitamin D, being extremely abundant in the body, has become a molecule used almost everywhere in the reactions and modulations of many parameters of the organism.

And as we moved north, we started to have problems: vitamin D was lacking.

We still carry these problems with us nowadays because it has only been a few thousand years since we emigrated, and evolutionary adaptation takes much longer than that.

One way to have an adequate amount of vitamin D in the blood would be to feed like the Eskimos by eating raw seals in large quantities.

Or we could expose ourselves to the sun for a long time and over large body surfaces every day.

However, these options are tricky enough to put in place ...

It is definitely easier to take vitamin D through supplementation.

One of the main problems we have with age is that the vitamin D in the body is decreasing more and more because it is needed more for various reasons; it is produced less and less, and usually, you make less outdoor life.

The result is that 70% of the elderly whose blood vitamin D concentration was checked were highly deficient.

With aging, it therefore becomes essential to integrate it because we have less and less, while the body requires more and more.

Vitamin D is essential in many processes related to the body's aging. One of the effects that has been noted is that vitamin D lengthens telomeres by activating telomerase.

A massive study examined the longest-lived people on Earth, those who live much longer and healthier, subjecting them to a whole series of research to see what they might have different in their bodies from the others.

One of the crucial things that has been noted is that all the longest-lived people on Earth have large amounts of vitamin D and Omega 3 in their blood.

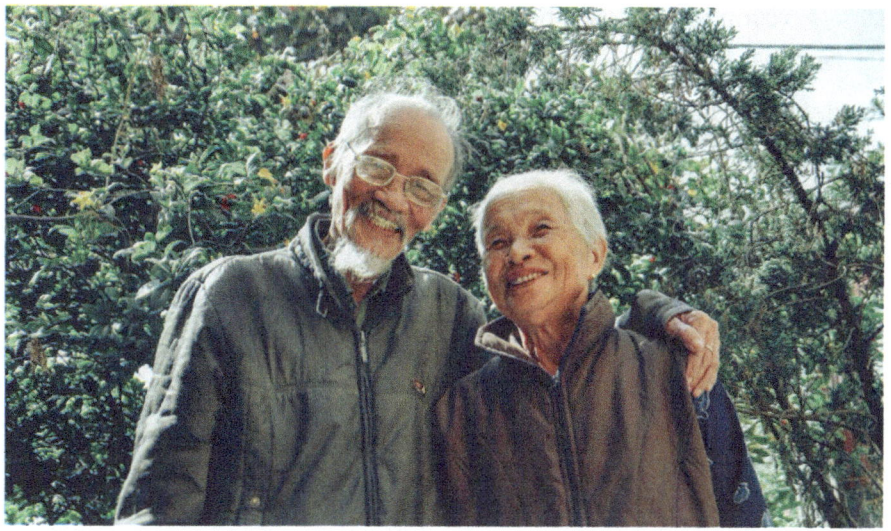

The medical sector generally recommends supplementing it only when a particular deficiency is found, not continuously, and with too low doses that, as we have seen, are ineffective.

Taking vitamin D occasionally, once a month or once a week, does not affect the average level in the blood.

It is therefore necessary to take it every day in rather large quantities, for long periods. No harmful side effects were detected except at extremely high levels.

Important: D3 (calciferol) should be chosen and not D2.

It is always to be taken together with vitamin K2 (or MK7).

DOSAGE: from 5,000 to 10,000 IU per day (for every 1000 IU of vitamin D3, associate 100 micrograms of K2).

How do you choose the dosage? It is necessary to carry out blood tests to detect the quantity of vitamin D present in our body.

Approximately:

- if the quantity detected is less than 20 ng/dl (or 50 nmol/l), we recommend doses between 8 and 10 thousand IU.
- if the quantity detected is around 30 ng/dl (or 75 nmol/l), we recommend doses between 6 and 8 thousand IU.
- if the quantity detected is around 50 ng/dl (or 125 nmol/l), we recommend doses between 5 and 8 thousand IU.
- if the quantity detected is around 80 ng/dl (or 200 nmol/l), we recommend doses of between 2 and 5 thousand IU.

NAD (NICOTINAMIDE ADENINE DINUCLEOTIDE)

NAD is involved in producing ATP (energy in the mitochondria) and DNA repair mechanisms.

Without ATP, the body has no energy; without energy, metabolic processes, and various physiological activities, starting with the immune system, do not work.

It is naturally produced in the body, starting with the amino acid tryptophan; after a processing elaboration, it is converted into the NAD substance, which is usable by the body, but the process is slow and therefore, as the demand for this type of molecule increases, the body begins to weaken.

NAD plays a fundamental role in DNA repair mechanisms; in practice, it acts as a "glue" in a series of chemical reactions that recover damaged DNA's functioning.

As we know, DNA is continuously damaged every day, so having a mechanism that repairs it is essential, as leaving the DNA unrepaired means that the cell is destined to stop working very soon.

With increasing age, these mechanisms become more and more critical, and therefore, NAD is increasingly in demand.

Practically, the NAD is halved, as available quantity, every 20 years of life, beginning from birth.

The substances that are precursors of NAD, needed by the body to synthesize it, are various forms of vitamin B3. such as nicotinic acid, nicotinamide, nicotinamide riboside and other similar substances.

A striking example of the problems that can arise as a result of the reduction of NAD in our body is a particular type of disease where the lack of NAD produces truly severe effects: pellagra.

Typically, pellagra is a disease that was caused in the past by a diet that was too low in vitamins, and produced a number of very adverse effects: diarrhea, dermatitis, dementia, and eventually death. For many years, the cure for pellagra has been drinking milk, but they didn't know why. It was then seen in 1937 that unpasteurized milk contains a large amount of nicotinamide: 60% nicotinamide and 40% nicotinamide riboside.

The simplest way to increase the amount of NAD is to provide the precursors from the outside. We find many supplements on the market that claim to deliver NAD.

Usually, what is found on the market is NAD+ (which is the active part of NAD, an oxidative agent that can accept electrons from other molecules).

There is also the option of delivering NAD with skin patches (very expensive), which deliver NAD directly and for a long time into the blood; this produces an increase in the detectable concentration, but it is not certain that everything ends up inside the cells.

NAD is a very large molecule, and therefore, it is likely that it will not be able to pass through the cell walls; thus, it is not said that increasing the quantity in the blood automatically increases the available amount inside the cells.

There are many supplements that you can take orally instead.

NAD can be generated from tryptophan, an amino acid, and other substances that are derivatives of vitamin B3 (Niacin).

When it comes to supplements, you'll often see just B3 or Niacin mentioned. But there's more to the story! There are several forms of B3, each with its own effects and benefits. For instance, nicotinic acid (often abbreviated as NA) is one type, while nicotinamide (NAM) is another. You might also come across nicotinamide riboside (NR) and nicotinamide mononucleotide (NMN). Each of these has unique properties that can impact your health in different ways.

In any case, these supplements always require a good presence of B3 vitamins and tryptophan in the diet; therefore, by inserting this type of NMN or NR supplements, the diet must be rich in vitamin B3 (contained in white meat, spinach, peanuts, beef liver, brewer's yeast and some fish such as salmon, swordfish, and tuna).

No side effects have been reported, so they are safe molecules to take; however, you have to be careful if you have had neoplastic diseases because NAD increases the energy level in all the body cells, so maybe even those you don't want to activate.

In any case, it is essential, before taking this type of supplement, **to consult with a doctor** who knows your medical history.

If you want to get the most, you can take supplements in particular formulations that produce the following effects: integration of precursors, reactivation of the recycling enzyme, and deactivation of the two subsequent enzymes that go into methylation and excessive consumption of NAD. These supplements can also be quite expensive.

Among the less expensive formulations, *riboside* is the one we recommend.

Recent studies have shown a better efficacy of NMN when combined with TMG (trimethylglycine), which, among other things, decreases plasma homocysteine levels (Homocysteine Test: MedlinePlus Medical Test, n.d.).

Warning: the "NMN + NR" supplements should be kept cool or, in any case, stabilized. Hence, it is necessary to verify that they have some kind of stabilization mechanism.

DOSAGE: 100-500 mg per day

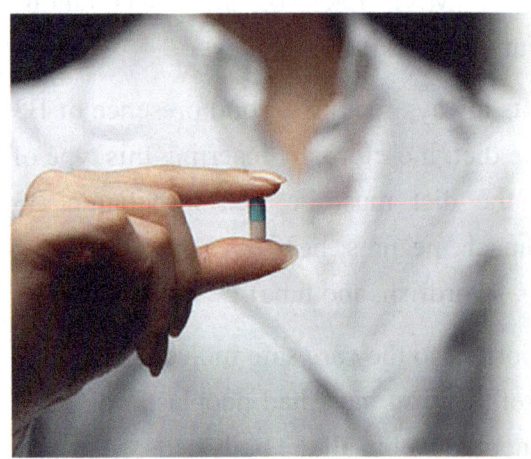

RAPAMICINA

RAPAMYCIN

Rapamycin is a drug used as an immunosuppressant to support transplants and coronary implants to prevent rejection in organ transplants.

The substance differs from other anti-aging drugs because it has a functioning mechanism that affects a protein called mTOR, which regulates cell growth.

One of the most exciting abilities of Rapamycin is that it induces autophagy.

Autophagy selects the quality parts of a cell, gets rid of the poor ones, and uses them as fuel to function better; therefore, it purifies, regenerates, and improves the cell simultaneously. It is the opposite trend to that involving diseases such as Alzheimer's and Parkinson's, in which cellular degeneration proliferates.

Specifically, it does this through TRPML1, which is found on the lysosome membrane and is a calcium ion channel.

In practice, if the TRPML1 channel is inactive, there is neurological degeneration; if the TRPML1 channel is stimulated, degeneration is fought.

A preponderance of evidence demonstrating the safety of Rapamycin in healthy humans has been well examined.

Since its approval by the FDA, Rapamycin has been used by millions of patients with very few mild and reversible side effects.

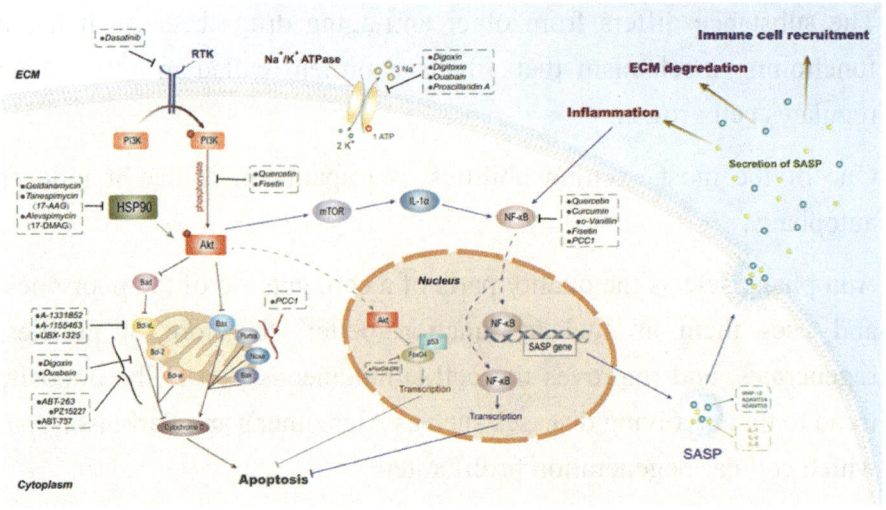

SENOLYTICS

Senolytics are molecules capable of eliminating senescent cells or at least reducing their secretory phenotype (anti-SASP effect).

SASP is the acronym for Senescence Associated Secretory Phenotype.

This biological phenomenon consists of the high secretion of pro-inflammatory and pro-oxidant factors by the aged cells, representing the main cause of their harmful effects.

From a biological point of view, SASP should act as a stimulus to prevent the proliferation of damaged cells and to solicit their immune neutralization. However, as we age, the dysfunctional evolution of the immune system promotes the accumulation of senescent cells and inhibits the function of stem cells.

A senolytic is a molecule, natural or synthetic, capable of selectively inducing the death of aged cells. Senolytic agents can target senescent cells through genetic or pharmacological approaches.

Considering the pro-oxidant and pro-inflammatory stimuli generated by aging cells, research on senolytics has turned towards natural substances with antioxidant and anti-inflammatory actions.

These include various polyphenols, which have long been studied as "anti-senescence" molecules:

Fisetin

Fisetin is a flavonol structurally and functionally related to quercetin. Fisetin has both senolytic and senomorphic activity, depending on the cell type.

It has been shown to extend mice's health and life span and reverse tissue damage when given to older animals. Fisetin is present in vegetables (onions and cucumbers), fruit (persimmons, apples, strawberries), wine, tea, and nuts, with concentrations ranging from 2 to 160 µg per gram.

Luteolin

Luteolin is another flavonoid of yellow color that is obtained from the plant *guaderella* (Reseda luteola). Food sources include celery, broccoli, artichokes, green pepper, parsley, thyme, dandelion, perilla, chamomile, carrots, olive oil, peppermint, rosemary, oranges, and oregano.

Piperlongumin

Piperlongumin is an alkaloid that abounds in the fruit of the Piper longum plant. Piperlongumin causes the selective killing of cancer cells by inhibiting the oxidative stress response proteins, which are important for the survival of cancer cells under high levels of reactive oxygen species (ROS). Also, in preliminary studies, piperlongumin has shown that it can preferentially kill senescent cells.

Tocotrienols

The accumulation of non-replicating cells in healthy tissues promotes the aging of the entire organism. Tocotrienols, which are members of the vitamin E family, have recently been shown to exert a dual action on healthy cells by stimulating natural growth, delaying senescence in cells, and arresting the growth of malignant cells.

These properties make Tocotrienols among the most promising senolytic compounds available.

Tocotrienols have also been shown to fight type 2 diabetes and metabolic syndrome, while delaying neurodegeneration.

A growing body of evidence in animal models demonstrates that the combination of Tocotrienols and Quercetin dramatically reduces blood levels of pro-inflammatory molecules.

As for the drugs we report:

Dasatinib is a drug used to treat some cases of leukemia. However, while Dasatinib and quercetin alone did not perform significant senolytic activities, their combination proved very active in this regard. The association between Dasatinib and quercetin also extended the span of health and life in elderly mice, improving cardiovascular function, and reducing frailty, neurological dysfunction, and bone loss.

Rapamycin (see dedicated chapter) is an immunosuppressant that decreases SASP and maintains cell cycle arrest, but does not kill senescent cells.

Metformin (see dedicated chapter) is a drug widely used for treating type 2 diabetes; it limits the activation of NF-κB, thus reducing the SASP.

Anakinra is a drug approved for use in cases of rheumatoid arthritis that reverses several effects of aging on the hematopoietic system (the hematopoietic system is the one in the body responsible for creating and generating new blood).

Finally, aspirin also showed mild anti-SASP effects.

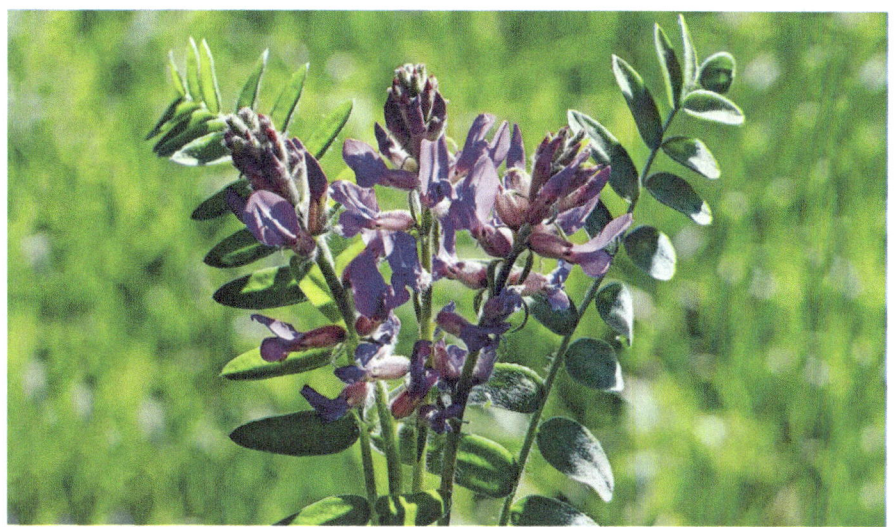

ASTRAGALUS

Recently, several studies have been performed on an extract from a plant used in traditional Chinese medicine since time immemorial, *Astragalus*, and it has been found that its active ingredient (cycloastrogenol) is able to increase telomerase by more than 25%.

Astragalus membranaceus (AM) is a medicinal herb that has shown immuno-regulatory properties in many infectious diseases.

Several studies have confirmed that it also has antiviral, anticancer, and cardiovascular protection functions.

Various studies on mice found that taking large doses of Astragalus increased glucose tolerance, bone density, and improved skin quality.

There was also an interesting study that found the positive effects of treatment with cycloastrogenol on the retina; other studies had previously seen a connection between telomeres length and macular degeneration due to aging.

Astragalus is a plant with countless properties, including antioxidant, anti-inflammatory, and immuno-modulating effects. It also improves sleep, memory, and the immune system.

It also has adaptogenic properties, as it lowers oxygen consumption in the mitochondria; finally, it supports the body's tolerance to stress.

Warning: there are more than two thousand species of Astragalus; only two have medical properties, and only one has these specific abilities that we have mentioned: the *Astragalus Membranaceus*.

DOSAGE: 500-800 mg of dry extract per day

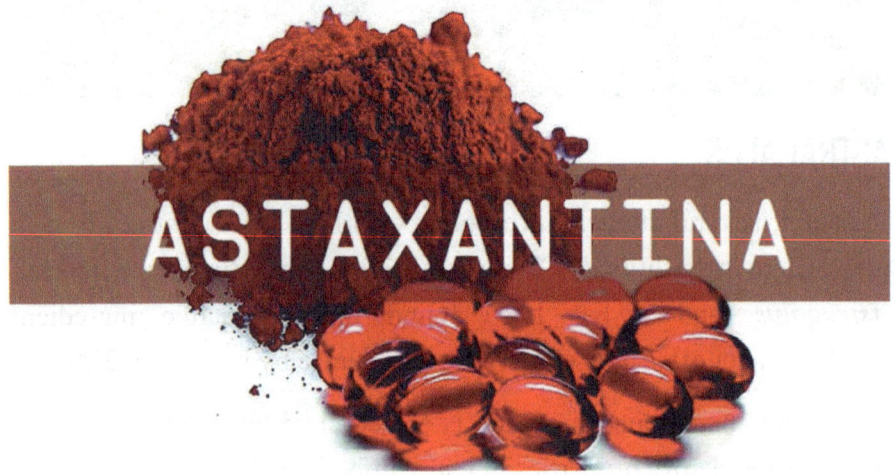

ASTAXANTHIN

Its name is *Haematococcus pluvialis,* and it is found mainly in Europe, Africa, North America, and part of India, wherever there are not very large quantities of water; it is a carotenoid naturally present in some algae.

When there are stressful conditions, individual cells begin to produce this substance, astaxanthin, which protects against cell breakdown.

In our body, it does exactly the same thing, so it protects us from various types of stress, such as oxidation stress and free radicals, so it acts as an anti-inflammatory and repairs cell damage.

In many studies, astaxanthin has been found to help control the sugar level in many people with diabetes. In other brain research, it was found that the administration of astaxanthin produced a reduction in neural degeneration.

In addition to fighting inflammation and free radicals, astaxanthin has also been shown to activate the immune system and T-type cells, inhibiting autoimmune reactions.

It also acts on the mucosal system, which is found both in the gastrointestinal and respiratory tract, and it is the first line of defense against any type of attack from the outside world, such as bacteria and viruses. In the cardiovascular system, astaxanthin lowers systolic blood pressure, improves the functioning of the heart, and helps prevent atherosclerosis and cardiovascular diseases.

In addition, a protective capacity of the retina was detected.

Astaxanthin acts in a much more powerful way than other antioxidants: it is 200 times more potent than polyphenols, 150 times more than anthocyanins, 75 times more than Alpha Lipoic Acid, 500 times more than vitamin E, 50 times more than beta-carotene.

DOSAGE: 10-40 mg per day

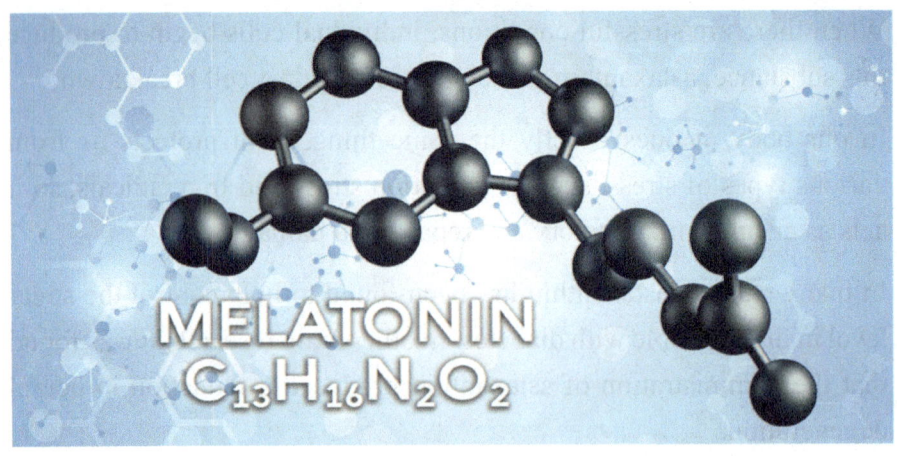

MELATONIN

Melatonin is a hormone that your body produces in a small gland at the base of your brain called the pineal gland. It acts on the hypothalamus and has the primary function of regulating the sleep-wake cycle, making sure you get the rest you need.

But melatonin does more than just help you sleep; it is also a cellular protector and antioxidant and is involved in a whole series of reactions to maintain the correct metabolic state. It protects cell membranes, mitochondria, and the cell nucleus.

It also regulates blood pressure, the physiology of the ovaries, and the immune system.

Melatonin administration has many positive effects on hyperglycemia, dyslipidemia, hyperinsulinemia, insulin resistance, and hypertension.

It is an epigenetic modifier.

DOSAGE: 2-4 mg per day, one hour before bedtime. No more than three times a week (to avoid addiction).

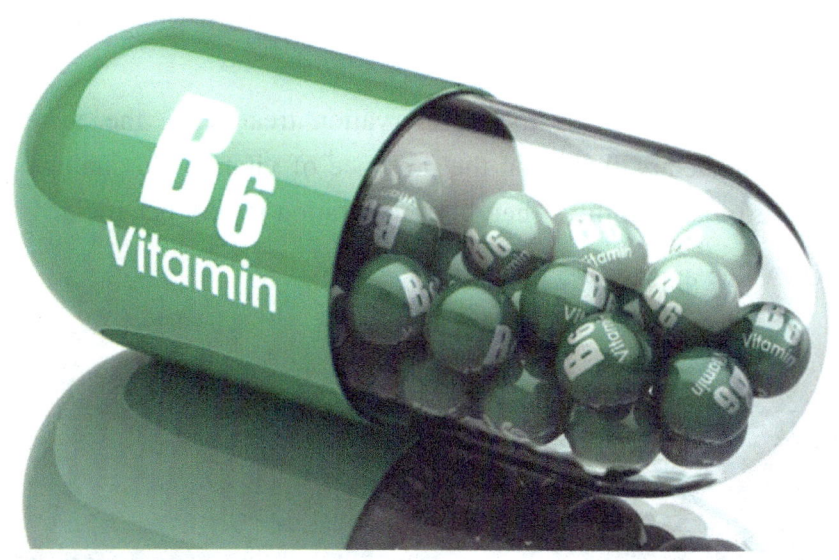

PYRIDOXINE (VIT B6)

Vitamin B6 has the fundamental role of constituting an immune barrier in defense against disease, stimulating brain functions, and preventing aging.

The A.G.E., which stands for Advanced Glycation End Products, is a substance that accumulates in the blood when there is an excess of glucose. There aren't many substances that can fight it; pyridoxine is one of the most effective.

The AGE is deposited in the arteries, producing arterial hardening, which in turn increases pressure. If we avoid this, the arteries remain elastic, and then we have better vascular health.

Clearly, not letting AGE deposit on collagen also helps to keep the skin elastic, so it has not only internal effects but also external ones.

Vitamin B6 (Pyridoxal phosphate) can be found in various foods, including wholemeal flour products (e.g., rye bread), rice, fruits such as avocados and bananas, hazelnuts, peanuts, sunflower seeds, wheat germ, brewer's yeast, fatty fish such as tuna and salmon, pork and chicken.

Some factors, such as food preservation treatments, the adsorbing power of dietary fiber, and the presence of vitamin B6 analogs, can limit its bioavailability. Therefore, integration is very beneficial.

DOSAGE: approx. 1.5 mg per day

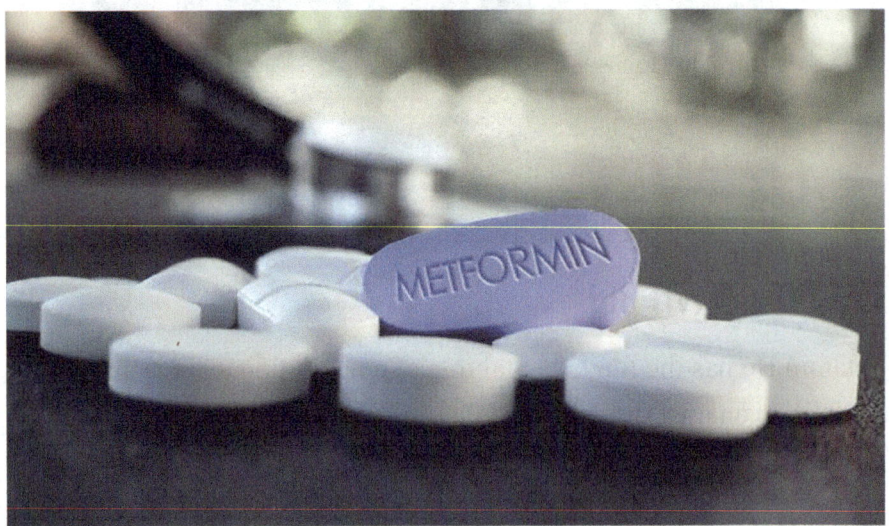

METFORMIN

Metformin is a substance that has been known for quite some time; it was developed for the treatment of diabetes and was used instead of insulin; for this reason, we have a vast knowledge of both the side effects (in specific doses and certain subjects it can also be dangerous) and the positive effects it can produce.

Subsequently, insulin treatment became predominant in the treatment of diabetes, and metformin was shelved due to the side effects that insulin does not have. Those effects are precisely those that interest us in slowing cell aging.

The main effects are a reduction of hyperglycemia (therefore, the excess of glucose in the blood), a reduction of the use of fatty acids, and a reduction of glucogenesis (i.e., the generation of new glucose).

Metformin also positively affects DNA methylation, therefore affecting how these substances are attacked and how they arrange themselves; moreover, it also appears to promote DNA repair capabilities.

Especially in conjunction with Resveratrol, it provides protection against DNA damage.

Very recently, it has been seen that metformin also has another significant effect in reducing inflammation: it inhibits the differentiation of monocytes into macrophages (different types of cells of the immune system), thus inhibiting cardiovascular problems, atherosclerosis, and insulin resistance.

Metformin also affects stem cells.

However, metformin blocks the metabolism of some vitamins, particularly vitamin B12, which must therefore be given as a supplement each time it is taken.

Metformin belongs to a class of drugs called "biguanides"; it is extracted from a plant called *Galega officinalis*—a plant that was already used in the Middle Ages as a remedy for the symptoms of diabetes.

This is a powerful drug that should only be taken with a medical prescription.

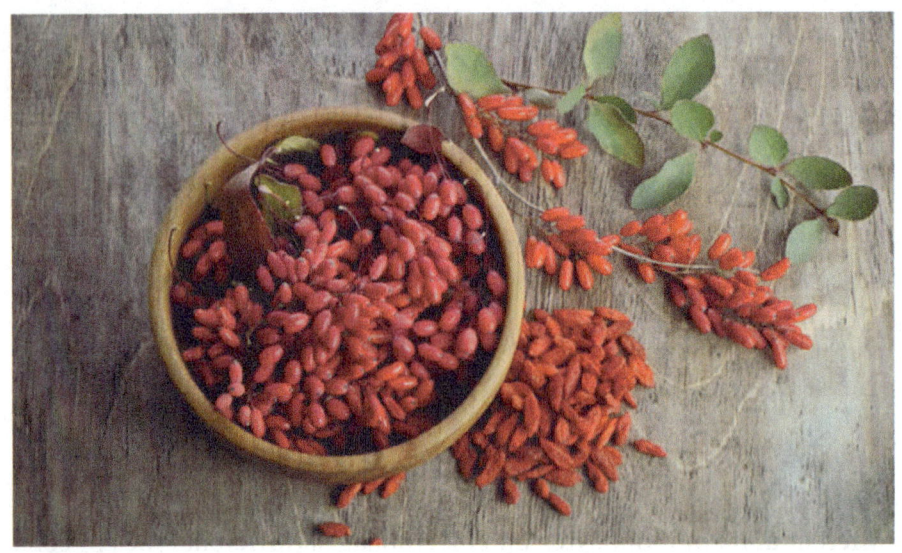

BERBERINE

Berberine is a fascinating alternative to metformin, and the best part is, you don't need a prescription to get it.

So, what is berberine? It's an alkaloid compound and is found in several plants: Hydraste, Cottide, Oregon grape, Barberry, and the Curcuma tree.

It has been used for millennia to fight infections; it has antibacterial and antifungal properties. Plus, it generally helps to boost the immune system's response.

Berberine has a metformin-like ability to reduce blood triglycerides and LDL (bad) cholesterol and increase HDL (good) cholesterol.

Recent studies have also shown a great hypoglycemic efficacy, i.e., the reduction of blood sugar, in patients who have type 2 diabetes mellitus; also, in this case, it seems that berberine acts at the level of receptors: it increases the expression of the receptors for insulin, therefore increases the sensitivity to this hormone, and reduces insulin resistance.

It also activates some metabolic pathways, in particular, AMPKinase, which is the process that breaks down fat deposits.

Like metformin, berberine also reduces telomeres shortening.

However, one good thing that metformin has and that it does not have berberine is that metformin has excellent bioavailability and absorbs well into the body; for berberine, on the other hand, the bioavailability is very low: 80% of what is absorbed is metabolized in the liver, produces no effect, and is discarded.

Therefore, it is necessary to take it three or four times a day, in order to ensure a more or less constant amount in the blood.

In a 2012 study, they gave several subjects 500mg of berberine three times a day; it was seen that in these subjects, the triglycerides levels were lowered, and cholesterol and even inflammatory factors were improved, without having side effects.

A 2015 study found that berberine counteracts the degeneration of neurons. It also appears that berberine can help with depression; not much research has been done in this area, but initial studies have seen that it increases the level of serotonin, dopamine, and norepinephrine.

DOSAGE: most studies have focused on a standard dose of 500 mg 3 times a day.

Always remember that these substances that act on glucose levels and cholesterol levels must be taken in any case after a medical consultation.

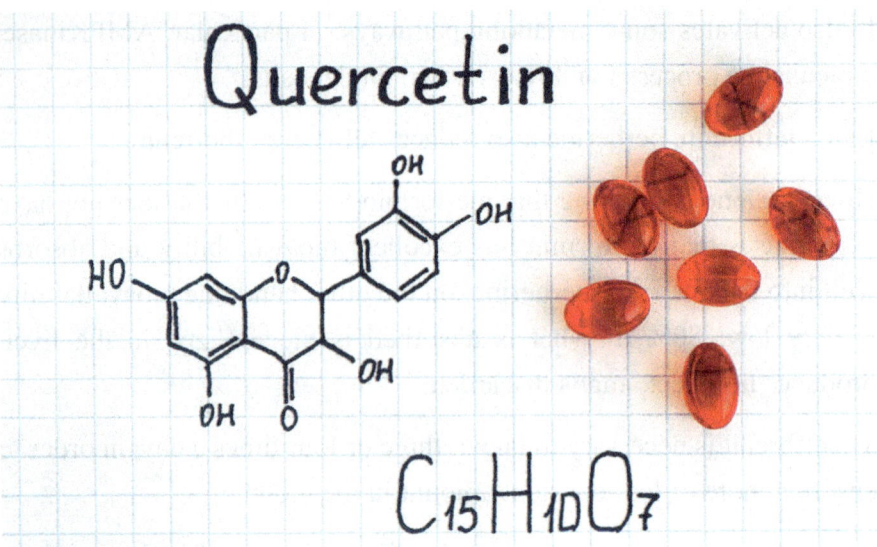

QUERCETIN

Quercetin is a polyphenol with potent anti-inflammatory, antioxidant, and immune-boosting effects.

Quercetin is found in capers (about 230 mg per 100 grams of capers), celery, cruciferous vegetables, and onions.

It is also present in some fruits such as apples (mainly in the peel), and also in black tea and white wine (unlike resveratrol, which is found mainly in red wine).

Quercetin is especially prescribed for allergies, asthma, arthritis, gout, hypertension, and neurodegenerative problems.

As with many other polyphenols, the effects are also positive on the cardiovascular systems, infections, inflammatory processes, diabetes, gastrointestinal tract function, and nervous system problems.

Quercetin appears to be one of the most potent flavonoids that protect the body against reactive oxygen species; however, one must be careful because, at high concentrations, it can become an oxidant itself.

Quercetin was found to block the release of histamines in the 1970s. Histamines are produced and then excreted by various cells to respond to stress, subsequently stimulating the inflammatory response.

Quercetin inhibits one of the enzymes responsible for the metabolization of Resveratrol in the liver, so the effects of Resveratrol are maintained for longer by taking it together with quercetin.

In a typical Mediterranean diet, about 30/40 mg of quercetin per day is taken through food, but several studies have shown that it takes at least 300 mg to see improvements from an anti-aging point of view.

DOSAGE: from 250 to 800 mg per day

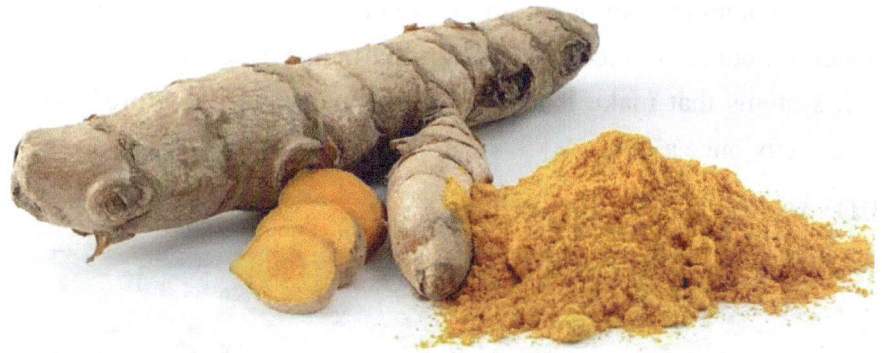

CURCUMIN

Curcumin is a polyphenol obtained from the root of *Curcuma longa* (turmeric).

The antioxidant and anti-inflammatory effect of curcumin is probably its most relevant property: it is an effect for which curcumin qualifies both as an inhibitor of the phenomena that trigger inflammation and as an interceptor of free radicals.

As we have seen, chronic inflammation is one of the leading causes of human aging; therefore, curcumin is one of the most effective substances for anti-aging treatments.

Curcumin, being lipophilic, can pass cell membranes, and this is important because it acts both inside the cells, in the cytoplasm (the liquid substance inside the cells), and in the inter-cellular liquid (that between one cell and another).

Curcumin makes up just 3% of the turmeric spice, so to get the effects we are discussing, we need to get supplements with the specific curcumin extract.

One problem with curcumin is that its blood concentration (bioavailability) peaks two hours after intake and is practically zero after four hours. Hence, it has a rather short half-life.

However, a number of preparations are now available on the market in which curcumin is incorporated into particular lysosomal structures, i.e., systems that make it available for longer and, therefore, can be taken only once a day.

DOSAGE: 500-1000 mg per day

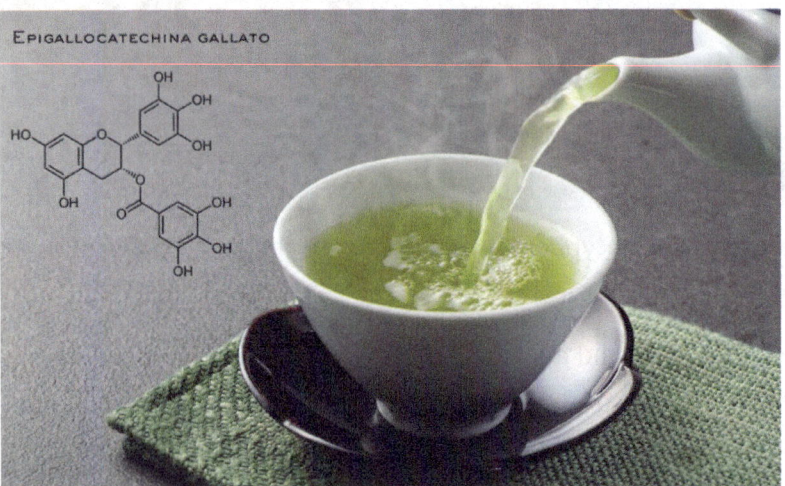

GREEN TEA

The EGCG (epigallocatechin gallate), the active substance of green tea, has many positive effects: first of all, it acts against reactive oxygen species, which, as we have seen, are very harmful to cells and metabolism. It is also an antioxidant and prevents tumor-like degeneration. It is a good anti-inflammatory and also has a robust effect against degeneration of the cardiovascular system.

Another interesting thing about green tea is its ability to activate AMPKinase, which we know to be extremely important for a whole series of metabolic reactions and the inhibition of metabolic alterations.

Earlier, we talked about how AGEs, which are byproducts of excess sugar, can be harmful. The great news is that green tea not only lowers the levels of AGEs in the body but also reduces their receptors, known as RAGE.

Many laboratory experiments on mice showed a substantial increase in cognitive and spatial abilities.

In other laboratory experiments on humans, a positive effect has been seen in contrasting senile dementia, Alzheimer's, and Parkinson's.

EGCG can be taken by drinking green tea, but for each cup of green tea, there is 70 to 90 mg of the active substance, while a supplement contains 400 to 600mg. We find it easier to take one tablet than a dozen cups of green tea daily.

It should also be noted that recent research, which requires further investigation by the European community, indicates a potentially negative effect on liver cells in concentrations above 800 mg per day; therefore, it is recommended that liver cells stay below this value.

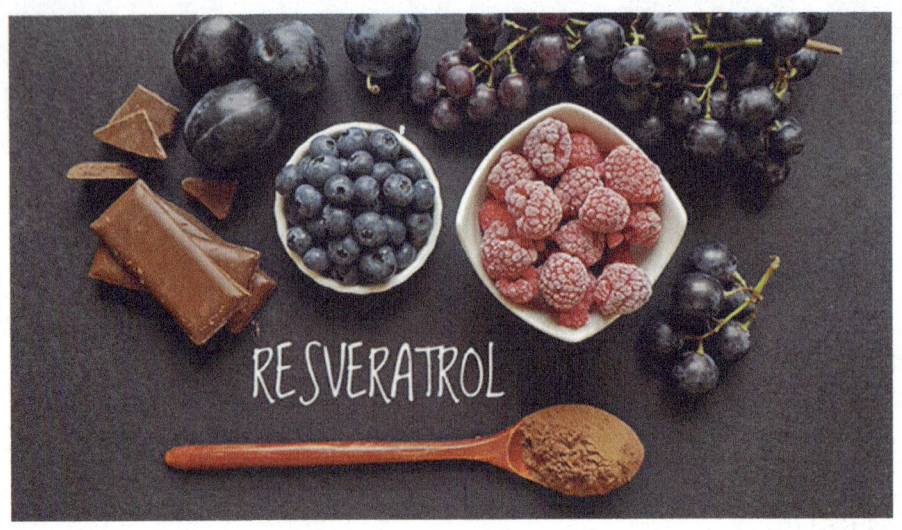

RESERATROL

Resveratrol is a non-flavonoid phenol that has been studied extensively in the anti-aging world. It is a substance that has been used for more than two thousand years in Ayurvedic medicine, as well as in traditional Chinese and Japanese medicine. It is extracted from plants endemic to East Asia, Japan, Korea, and China.

Resveratrol is mainly found in grapes, especially in the skin—red wine contains much more than white wine. You can also find it in other fruits like blueberries, currants, and peanuts. Because resveratrol is lipophilic, it can easily penetrate cell membranes and work directly inside cells, which is why it is so effective.

The problem is that it is metabolized very quickly. Therefore, its bioavailability (i.e., how long it maintains a concentration sufficient to act in the organism) is very short. Nonetheless, it can do very beneficial things in that short period.

The resveratrol molecule is made up of two phenolic rings connected by two carbon connections. These carbon links can be of the *cis* or *trans* type. The *trans* version has been found to be highly more effective; for this reason, on the market, we often find that version of resveratrol which is preferred over the others.

The most significant anti-aging effect of resveratrol is that it activates telomerase.

Another intriguing effect of resveratrol is that it activates AMP Kinase (Adenosine Mono Phosphate-Kinase). This process is vital for certain gene activities, for DNA repair, and for DNA metabolism itself.

Another significant effect is on stem cells, especially mesenchymal ones; this promotes bone production, which is extremely important in preventing all degenerations that have to do with the skeletal system caused by advancing age.

Glucose control is another substantial effect of resveratrol (hence improving insulin sensitivity).

It has also been seen in several studies that it promotes the activity of dental stem cells.

Laboratory mice treated with resveratrol showed an improvement in almost all morphological structures in their neurons; therefore, more connections, dendrites, and axons worked better and with more interconnections.

In experiments carried out on monkeys, it was seen that treatments with resveratrol caused a substantial increase in cognitive abilities and skills, therefore linked to evolved brain capacities.

Positive effects were also seen on the eyes: resveratrol has been shown to be effective in macular degeneration, delaying or even preventing it, a decline that seems inevitable with age. The same can be said for the crystalline lens.

The problem with resveratrol is that it is not very bio-available, and its half-life is very short: 70 percent of what is ingested is rapidly degraded by the liver, and it is still available for a period ranging from 30 up to a maximum of 180 minutes. To solve these problems, a "relative" of resveratrol, called *pterostilbene*, has been brought into existence.

Pterostilbene is a resveratrol molecule where a hydroxyl group has been replaced with a methoxy group, thus producing a somewhat different molecule while having the same properties.

The crucial thing about pterostilbene is its longer bioavailability and its resistance to being metabolized and thus eliminated, so it is better to prefer preparations that contain pterostilbene rather than resveratrol.

A study has shown that compared to resveratrol, in equivalent doses, pterostilbene is a much more powerful modulator of cellular stress than its demethylated counterpart. A growing number of studies show that pterostilbene has beneficial effects on lipid and glucose metabolism, with a consequent improvement in insulin sensitivity.

A study conducted in mouse models with diabetes found that the effects of pterostilbene can be considered comparable to the experimental results of 500 mg/kg of oral metformin.

DOSAGE: 100 – 200mg

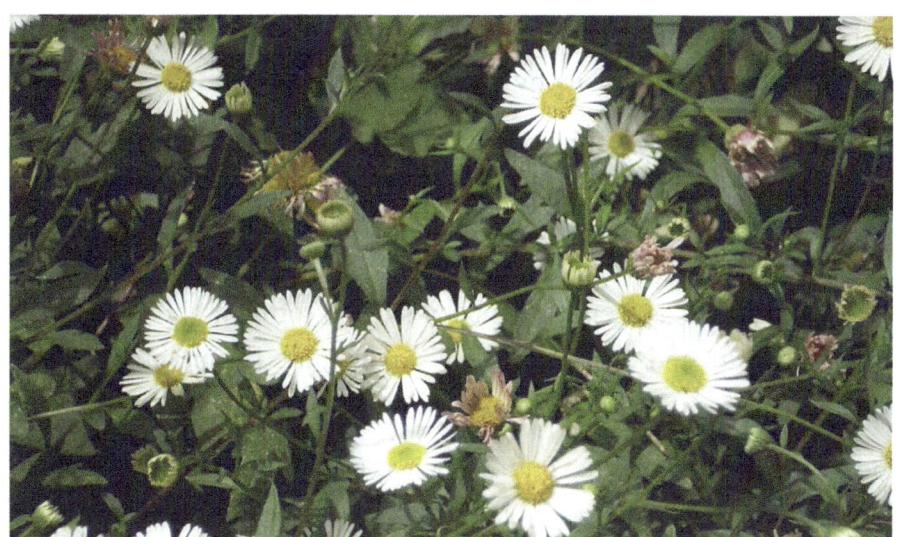

APIGENIN

Apigenin is a flavone present in celery leaves, parsley, and chamomile and is the aglycone of numerous natural glycosides, such as rhoifolin and isovitexin.

Research on apigenin has observed various properties: anti-inflammatory, antioxidant, anticancer, antibacterial, and antiviral.

Apigenin is also present in reasonable concentrations in yarrow, tarragon, coriander, echinacea, licorice, flax, passionflower, horehound, and spearmint. It has also been identified as an active ingredient in various other medicinal plants, including *Scutellaria barbata* (Lamiaceae), *Castanea sativa* (Fagaceae), *Portulaca oleracea* (frate grass), *Combretum erythrophyllum* (Combretaceae) and *Aquilegia oxysepala*, as well as in propolis.

Apigenin binds to some brain receptors (those of benzodiazepines), which can reduce anxiety and improve sleep quality.

In a study in mice, apigenin improved the depression caused by cortisol treatments.

It has been shown that apigenin and two of its glycosides exert anti-diabetic effects in the body by enhancing the cellular insulin response.

Apigenin can also lower blood fats and improve liver health.

In mice, it improved skin barrier function, promoting the growth of skin cells and the production of fat molecules and antimicrobial proteins.

Flavones such as apigenin have been studied for their ability to lower blood pressure and cholesterol levels, which are important indicators of heart disease risk.

It has been shown that flavonoids such as apigenin delay the decline in testosterone levels caused by aging in men. In particular, it has been noted that apigenin modifies a receptor (TBXA2) in the testes and the activity of an enzyme (aromatase) involved in the synthesis and metabolism of testosterone.

DOSAGE: 3 8 mg per kg of body weight per day

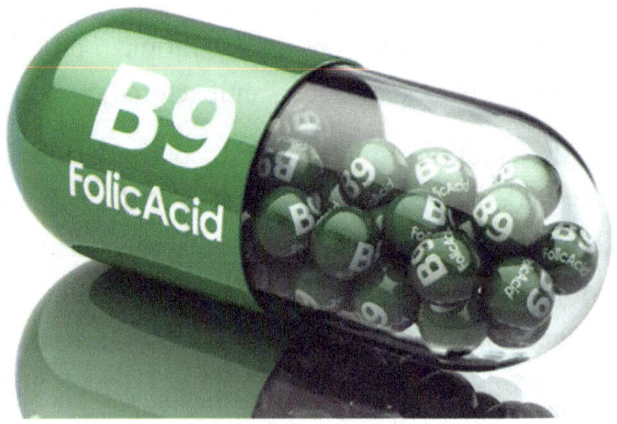

FOLIC ACID

Folic acid (vitamin B9) is important for epigenetics because it is necessary for the remethylation of homocysteine, a key chemical reaction of the metabolic pathway that synthesizes S-adenosyl methionine, the methyl donor group of histones, and reactions of DNA methylation.

It is essential for synthesizing proteins and forming hemoglobin and is particularly important for tissues undergoing proliferation and differentiation processes.

The amount of folate intake in the diet can be associated with the epigenetic state of the organism. Dietary folate deficiencies cause numerous health alterations that are most noticeable when they occur during embryonic development. In rats, maternal protein restriction during pregnancy leads to a loss of methylation of the gene promoter associated with glucose metabolism in the offspring.

Foods naturally rich in folate are green leafy vegetables (spinach, broccoli, asparagus, lettuce), legumes (beans, peas), fruit (kiwis, strawberries, and oranges), and dried fruit (such as almonds and walnuts).

As for foods of animal origin, liver, and other offal have a rather high folate content, as do some cheeses and eggs. However, it must be borne in mind that the process of preparing, cooking, and storing food can destroy a large part of the folate present in food, since these are water-soluble vitamins, sensitive to heat, light, air, and acidity.

For this reason, integration can be helpful.

DOSAGE: 0.2 0.4 mg per day

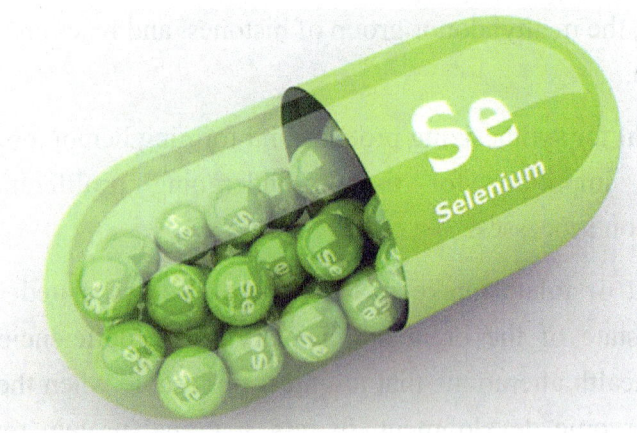

SELENIUM

Selenium is a non-metal chemical that is similar to sulfur and tellurium.

It is a substance that can modify an organism's epigenetic state at the DNA methylation and histone modification level.

Inside the cells, selenium allows the cellular antioxidants to function well. Being part of dozens of proteins, it also participates in various other processes, from DNA synthesis to the metabolism of thyroid hormones, through protection against infections and reproduction.

Selenium deficiency can reduce skeletal muscle function, interfere with red blood cell production, change skin and hair pigmentation, and increase nail brittleness. It can also predispose to disease in the presence of additional stresses such as viral infections, and can be associated with male infertility.

The most selenium-rich foods are fish and Brazil nuts. Other good sources are red meat, dairy products, and cereals.

In general, however, the amount of selenium present in foods of plant origin depends on the soil characteristics in which they were grown.

DOSAGE: 40 50 micrograms

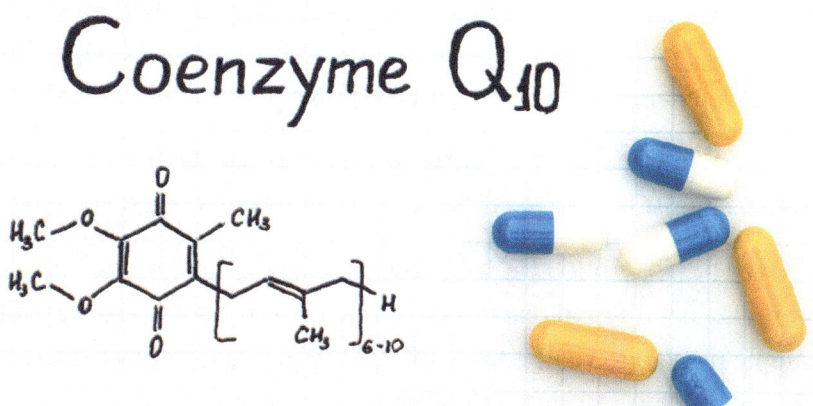

Q10

Coenzyme Q10 (ubiquinol) is a molecule present throughout the body and is particularly abundant in the heart, liver, kidneys, thyroid, spleen, and pancreas.

Coenzyme Q10 is essential for the proper functioning of many organs and for carrying out numerous chemical reactions in the body. Similar to a vitamin, it is a lipophilic molecule (insoluble in water) belonging to the group of coenzymes Q and exerts an antioxidant action. It is lacking in the presence of some pathologies.

Its intake is proposed against cardiovascular problems, diabetes, Parkinson's, muscular dystrophy, chronic fatigue syndrome, Lyme disease, Huntington's disease, and breast cancer.

It is also used to increase energy and resistance to physical exertion and to strengthen the immune system.

The powerful antioxidant role of coenzyme Q10, effective in controlling the peroxidation of membrane lipids and atherogenic LDL cholesterol particles, seems to be the main focus on which its clinical use insists.

By virtue of this activity, coenzyme Q10 is successfully used in the prevention of heart disease, in the prevention of hypertension, and associated damage, in the prevention and management of neurodegenerative diseases, and the prevention of cellular aging.

Recent works would also attribute to coenzyme Q10 a myoprotective action against oxidative stress elicited by physical exercise.

However, absorption is very slow: only 2-4% of the ubiquinone introduced with food reaches the bloodstream. With the intake of a Q10 supplement (three daily doses of 100 mg per day), it has been seen that the amount present in the lipoproteins is acceptable.

DOSAGE: 100 300 mg per day

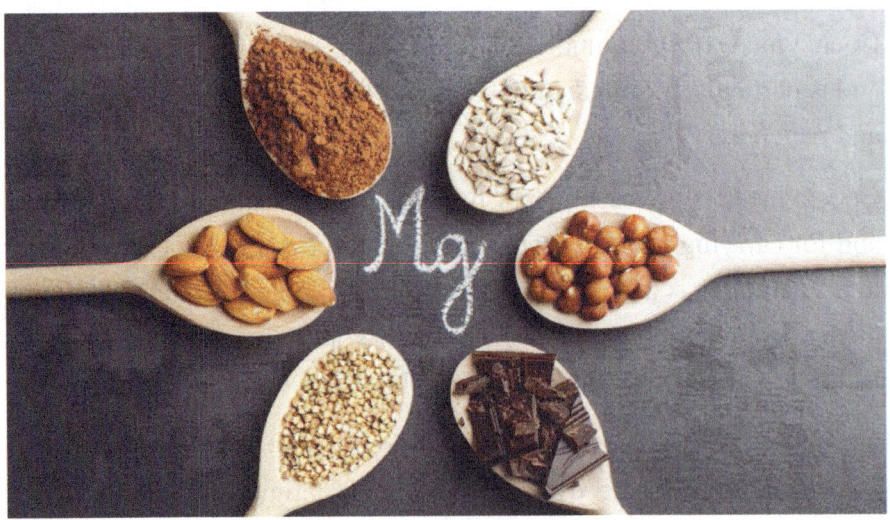

MAGNESIUM

As a quantity, magnesium is the fourth among the minerals present in our body and is essential for our health.

Magnesium is necessary for more than 300 biochemical reactions that take place in our body, and, among other functions, it contributes to normal muscle and nerve function, regulates the heartbeat, keeps the immune system efficient, and strengthens bone tissue.

It also contributes to regulating blood glucose levels and normalizing blood pressure, and is involved in energy metabolism and protein synthesis.

If you have sufficient magnesium supplies in the body, you are better protected from cardiovascular disease and dysfunctions in the immune system.

The overall health of the digestive system and kidneys influences magnesium stores significantly: magnesium is absorbed by the intestine and then transported by the blood to the cells and tissues of the body.

Many people with type 2 diabetes have low magnesium levels in their blood (hypomagnesemia). When magnesium is low, it can actually worsen insulin resistance.

Leafy green vegetables, such as spinach, are a good source of magnesium. Some legumes (such as beans and peas), some types of nuts (such as almonds), seeds, and whole grains also contain considerable quantities: non-whole grains, on the other hand, have a relatively low content.

As we age, our body's demand for magnesium increases considerably; in these cases, supplementation is helpful, if not necessary.

DOSAGE: 300 500 mg per day

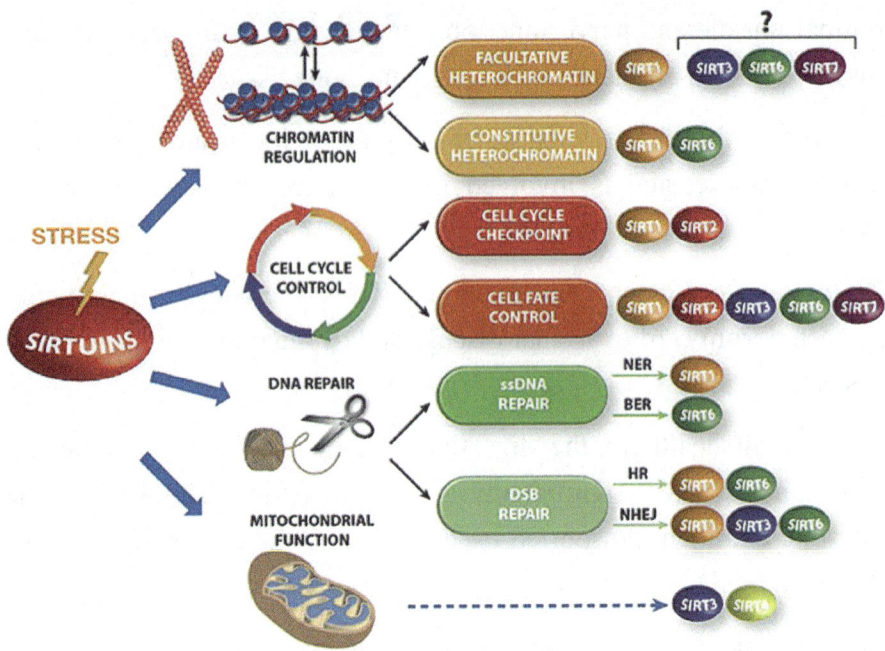

SIRTUINS

Sirtuins are proteins produced physiologically by our body, capable of performing various functions. In particular, these proteins slow down cellular aging and have the ability to intervene in metabolism.

Sirtuins activate energy consumption processes, drawing from fat reserves and obtaining energy from excess fat. They also protect cells from metabolic stresses and regulate the aging process. They are important indicators of the metabolic state, as they are produced when there is a shortage of nutrients.

Sirtuins are activated in fasting conditions. In the modern era, Western men never encounter periods of food shortages. However, our genetic make-up reminds us that several centuries ago, it was frequent to face periods of fasting, so it is still programmed to handle periods of severe nutrient scarcity.

How does this happen? By drawing from your own fat reserves and consuming excess fat. Therefore, weight loss is the consequence of activating the so-called *lean gene*.

By *lean gene*, we mean a specific family of genes called SIRT, which encodes sirtuins.

Recent studies and research have identified several substances capable of activating SIRT genes. These compounds, called STACs (SirTuin Activating CompoundS), signal the body to start the same metabolic processes obtainable with fasting. These are mainly made up of polyphenols, substances found naturally in many foods.

Daily consumption of these SIRT foods puts the lean gene into action. In this way, the synthesis of sirtuins is activated, favoring the consumption of excess fat mass.

SIRT foods are bitter cocoa, extra virgin olive oil, red wine, red onion, matcha tea, capers, celery, soy, strawberries, nuts, turmeric, buckwheat, kale, parsley, and arugula.

There are supplements on the market that stimulate the production of sirtuins.

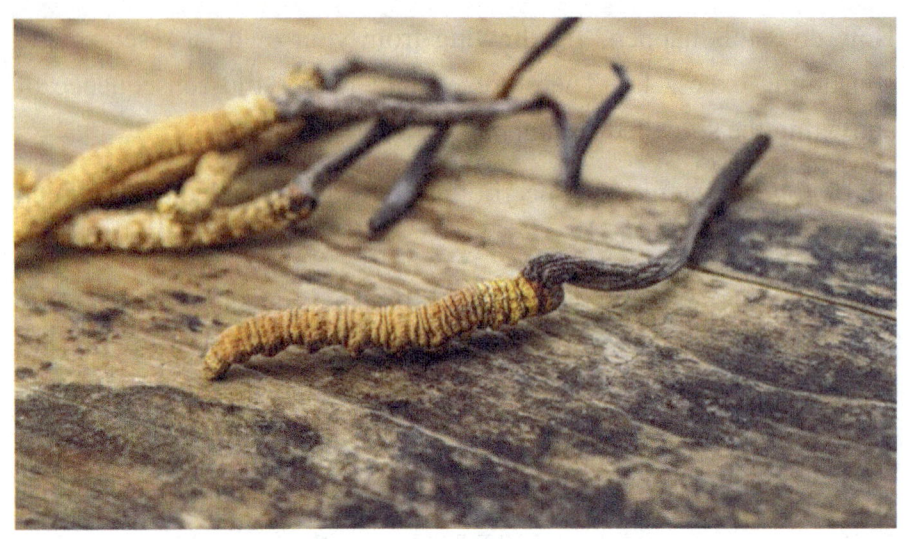

CORDYCEPS SINENSIS (*YARTSA GUNBU*)

Cordyceps Sinensis is a fascinating mushroom that originates from China. Chinese medicine says it can boost your immune system and is also considered an adaptogen, which means it can help increase the energy available to the body, which generally helps you manage stress.

Reduces total cholesterol and increases HDL cholesterol; improves physical performance, especially in states of stress; it has a hepatoprotective effect, with potential implications not only preventive but also therapeutic in the presence of viral hepatitis, hepatic steatosis, liver fibrosis, and liver cirrhosis; has an anti-hypertensive effect, with increased cardiovascular health; it can help in the presence of myocardial ischemia, atherosclerosis, and related diseases.

Improves kidney function; balances blood sugar by lowering blood glucose levels; modulates the sleep-wake cycle in the presence of difficulty falling asleep, thanks to a possible sedative effect on the central nervous system.

The chemical analysis of Cordyceps highlights an excellent lipid content (58% of unsaturated fats, especially linoleic and oleic, and 42%

of saturated fats), proteins, trace elements, vitamins, and polysaccharides.

At least two substances have been identified as notable active constituents; we are talking about cordycepin (structurally very similar to D-mannitol) and cordycepic acid (structurally similar to 3-deoxyadenosine).

Equally important in determining the pharmacological activities of Cordyceps seems to be its polysaccharide component, in which galactomannan abounds.

Other bioactive compounds include nucleosides (adenosine, guanosine, and uridine) and phytosterols (ergosterol, an important precursor of vitamin D).

Finally, among metals, elements such as zinc, magnesium, and manganese abound, which, from a physiological point of view, are very important for the development and maintenance of the gonads.

The published studies seem to confirm the properties of Cordyceps, in particular its immunomodulatory and antitumor effect, hypoglycemic, antihypertensive, promoter of hepatic, cardiac, and renal function and health, anti-aging, hypocholesterolemic, regulator of the sleep-wake cycle, antitussive, expectorant and antiasthmatic.

DOSAGE: 500 1000 mg per day

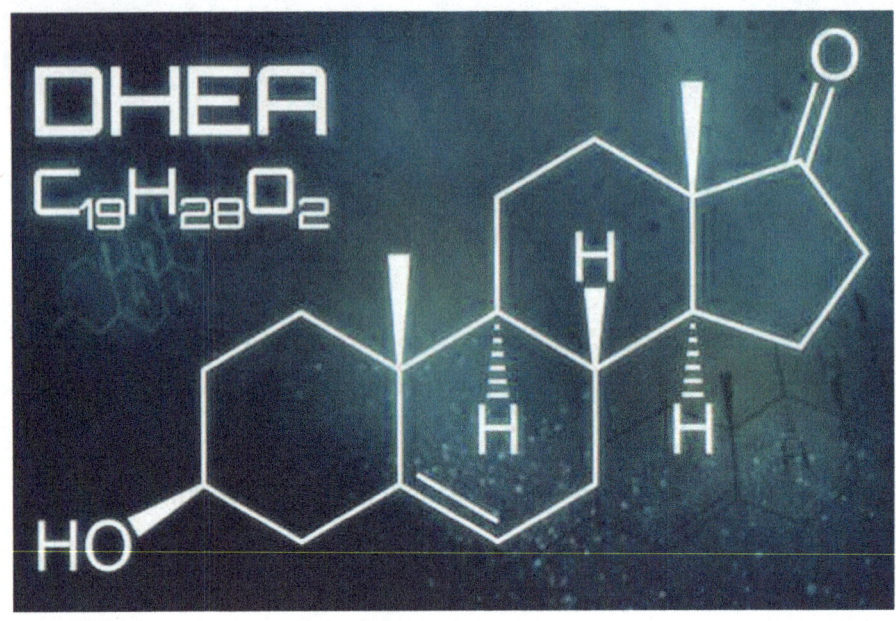

DHEA (DEHYDROEPIANDROSTERONE)

5-dehydroepiandrosterone is an endogenous natural steroid hormone. It is the primary steroid hormone produced by the secretion of the adrenal glands; it is also produced in the gonads and brain. DHEA is the most abundant circulating steroid in humans.

It is called the *hormone of youth* because it is the one that most of all decreases with age, already from the age of 30, in both men and women.

It has an indirect action because, in turn, it gives rise to other hormones (e.g., estrogen and testosterone) and a direct one, mainly on the nervous system.

DHEA has been shown to improve energy, body composition (increases lean and muscle mass), dryness (hair, skin, and vagina), sexuality, mood, depression, osteoporosis, fertility, skin-aging, the stress reaction, the immune system, as well as having a general anti-aging action.

DHEA can be used in various forms: micronized oral tablets, liposomal gel, cream, and vaginal suppositories. It is generally dosed in the blood as DHEA's (sulfate form of DHEA), which is more stable but can also be dosed in saliva.

DOSAGE: 50 200 mg per day

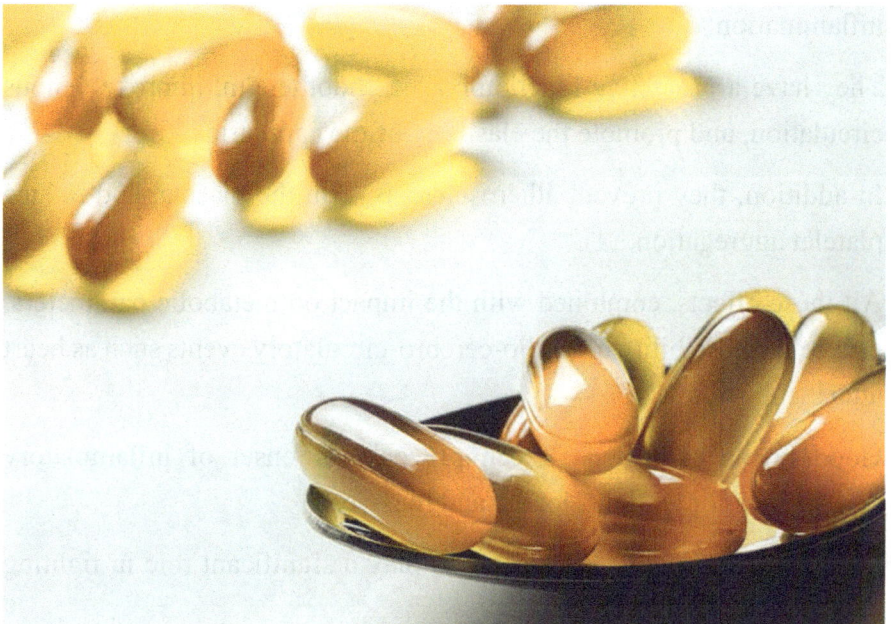

OMEGA 3

Omega 3s are polyunsaturated fats considered essential. In particular, their precursor (alpha-linolenic acid, ALA) cannot be synthesized by the body and, therefore, must be taken via food.

Essential fatty acids have a positive effect on lipemia.

Omega 3s mainly reduce triglycerides, while Omega 6s mainly improve cholesterol profile.

Omega 3s have a very positive role in dyslipidemias triggered or aggravated by type 2 diabetes mellitus. In addition to dyslipidemias, they also have a beneficial role in certain lesions due to chronic hyperglycemia.

They reduce blood pressure in people with primary arterial hypertension.

They are anti-inflammatory and lower the condition of systemic inflammation.

They have a protective function on the endothelium, improve venous circulation, and promote the elasticity of the capillaries.

In addition, they prevent atherosclerosis, thin the plasma, and reduce platelet aggregation.

All these effects, combined with the impact on metabolic parameters, reduce the possibility of cardio-cerebro-circulatory events such as heart attack and stroke.

Good levels of Omega 3 can prevent the onset of inflammatory discomforts for tendons, joints, and muscles.

Omega 3s, especially EPA, seem to play a significant role in fighting certain types of depression.

NB: Omega 3 in capsules oxidize easily, so keep them cool and dark. As an alternative to capsules, take fish oil in liquid form in glass containers.

DOSES: 2-5 g per day (of which at least 1-2 g of EPA)

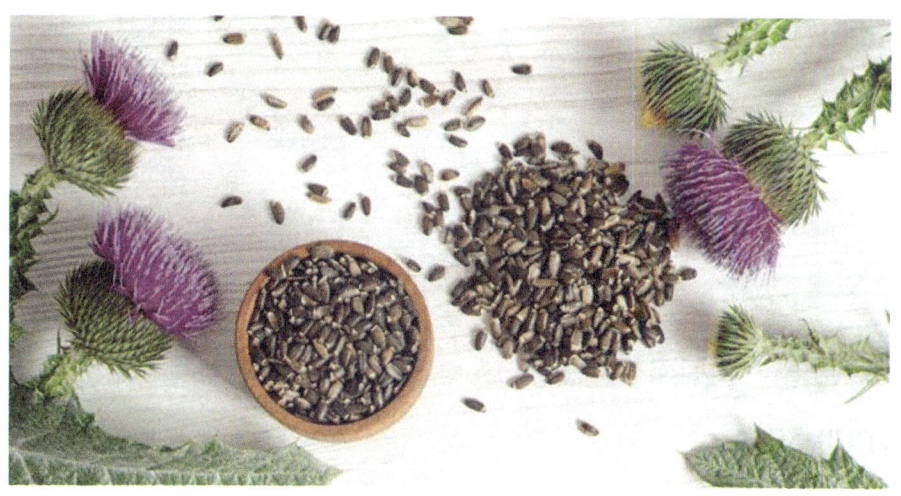

SILYMARIN

Silymarin is a mixture of silybin, silicristin, and silydianin (in the ratios of 3: 1: 1 respectively), three active ingredients found in different plants, including *Silybum marianum* (milk thistle).

Silymarin is a compound with important protective properties for the liver: in particular, it would be able to protect liver cells from inflammation and damage caused by oxidative stress and, at the same time, enhance the synthesis of liver proteins.

DOSAGE: 200 400 mg per day

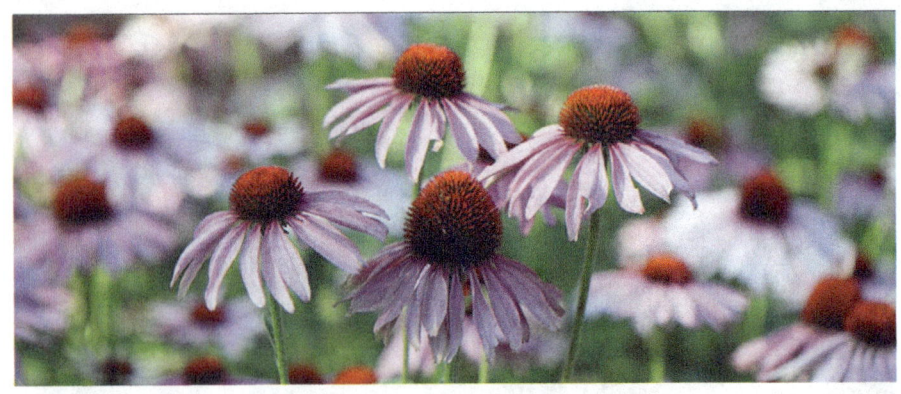

ECHINACEA

Echinacea is a plant with numerous properties, among which the anti-inflammatory, antibacterial, antiviral, and immunostimulating ones stand out.

Its antiviral and immunostimulating properties are due to glycoproteins and alkylamines, but above all, to the group of polysaccharides (arabinogalactans and arabinoxylans). The essential oil, rich in terpenes, is responsible for its antibacterial properties.

Therefore, we can say that echinacea's primary properties are to stimulate and strengthen the immune system especially against colds bacteriostatic, virustatic, and anti-inflammatory.

For external use, echinacea appears to exhibit skin-purifying properties, and some studies claim that it may be helpful in exerting an anti-wrinkle action.

DOSAGE: 400 500 mg per day

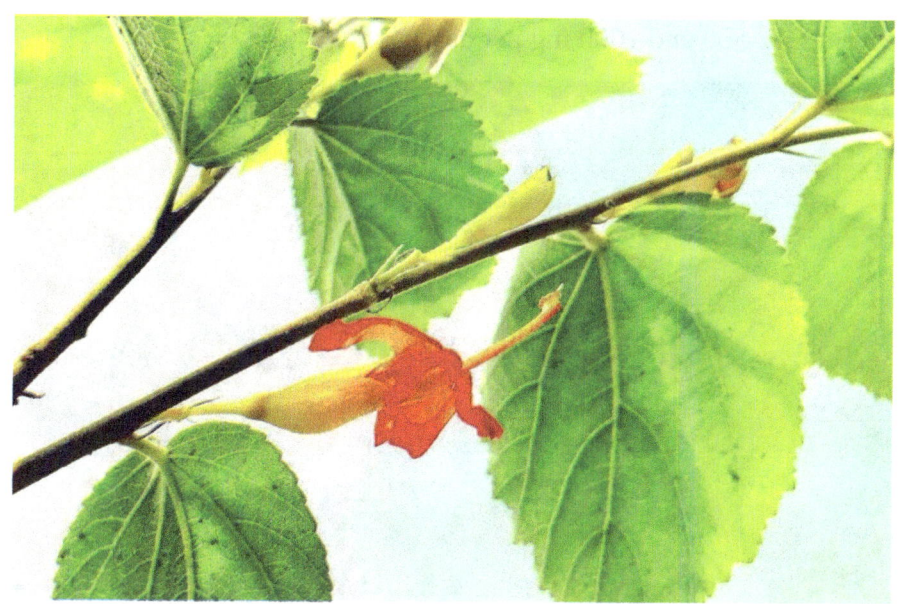

GYMNEMA SYLVESTRE

Gymnema Sylvestre is a plant known in traditional Ayurvedic medicine.

The anti-diabetic therapeutic virtue ascribed to the Gymnema phytocomplex deserves to be explored.

First of all, it should be noted that Gymnema extract is successfully used in the treatment of insulin-independent diabetes mellitus (type 2): it is believed that the active ingredients of Gymnema exert their action by roughly tracing the same mechanism of action of the drugs of synthesis with oral hypoglycemic activity (class: sulfonylureas).

In other words, the Gymnema phytocomplex is able to reduce plasma glucose levels by stimulating the pancreatic secretion of insulin (action in the beta cells of the pancreas).

The activity exerted in the pancreas could, in turn, protect the aforementioned pancreatic cells and, at the same time, favor their regeneration.

DOSAGE: 500 and 1000 mg per day

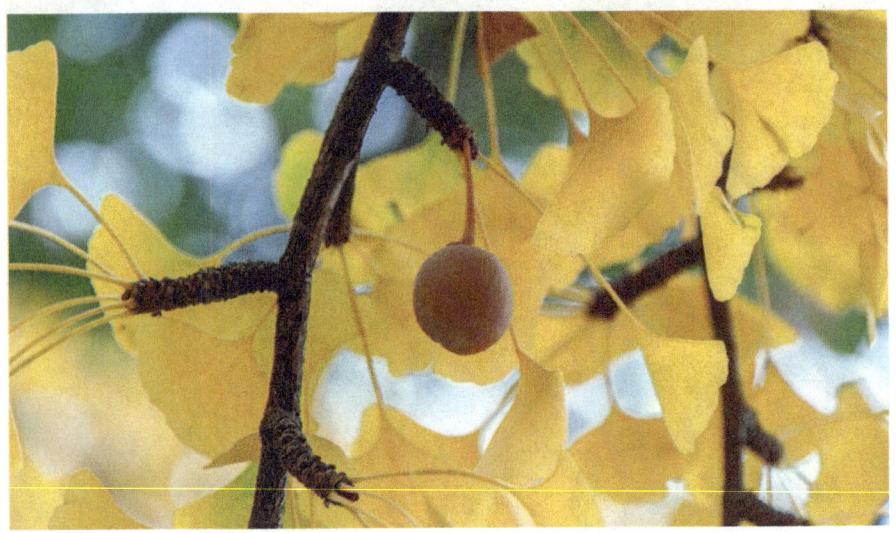

GINKGO BILOBA

Ginkgo Biloba is a gymnosperm plant, the only surviving species of the Ginkgoaceae family. It is an ancient tree whose origins date back 250 million years ago, and for this reason, it is considered a living fossil.

Ginkgo Biloba is used for memory disorders and conditions that are associated with reduced blood flow to the brain.

It also finds use in other problems associated with circulation disorders.

It is used in the case of cognitive problems associated with Lyme disease or depression, sexual dysfunction, glaucoma, diabetic retinopathy, and age-related macular degeneration.

Ginkgo Biloba is taken orally in the form of leaf extract or, less often, seed extract. The dosage and duration of administration depends on the problem you want to treat and can vary greatly from person to person.

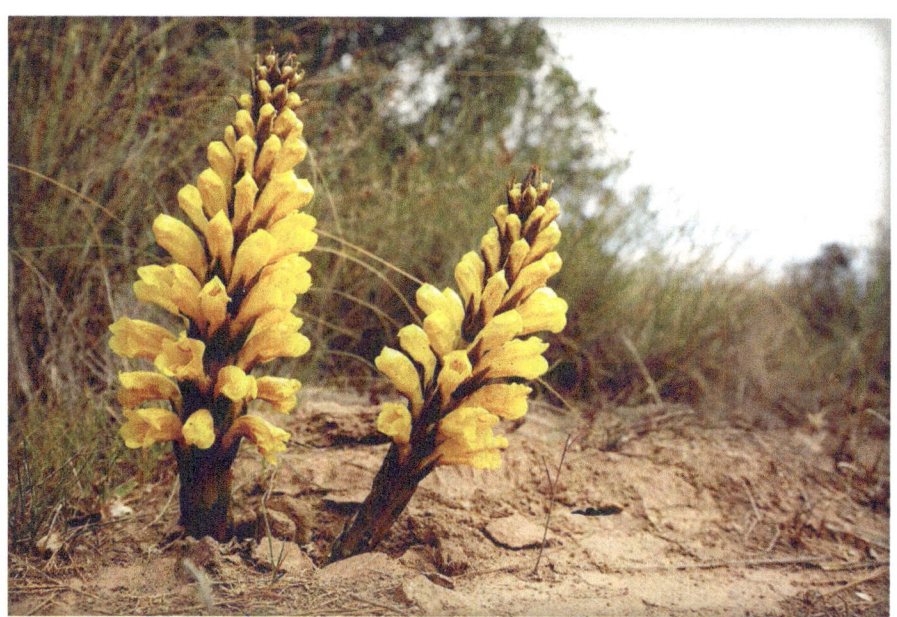

CISTANCHE DESERTICOLA

The Cistanche Deserticola is a very resistant type of perennial plant, from 30 cm to one and a half meters tall. It has thick, fleshy stems, and very large yellow flowers are produced at the top of the plant.

The Cistanche is a very particular form of life: it has no chlorophyll, so it is not green; it takes everything it needs to live by parasitizing on other plants; therefore, it is a plant called holoparasite, practically a parasite of everything, right from the roots.

The plant in Chinese is called Rou Cong-Rong because its main stem has a rather fleshy consistency (Rou), and its effects are calming (Cong-Rong). It is also called "desert ginseng". This plant has been used for more than two thousand years in traditional Chinese medicine, and is used to strengthen Yin and enhance Qi.

What this plant does: reduces the speed of aging, strengthens Yin, which is the male vital energy, and has also been used for a number of other effects: to cure constipation, to give virile potency, to cure diseases kidneys, to treat tetanus and also to reduce work fatigue.

Cistanche appears to have positive effects on telomeres. Cistanche polysaccharides increase telomerase activity in the heart and brain, in lymphocytes and macrophages; acteoside, which is one of the phenylethanoid glycosides found in Cistanche, is also able to increase the activity of telomerase in cardiac and brain tissue.

Cistanche recovers and removes various free radicals: it does so by removing them directly, blocking their production, and regulating the antioxidant enzymes that are linked to the metabolism of free radicals.

It has nine different substances that activate this free radical removal functionality; it improves and increases the production of endogenous antioxidants, i.e., antioxidant substances that the body normally produces on its own. For example, it increases the levels of mitochondrial glutathione, and in many other studies, it has been seen that it increases superoxide dismutase.

Furthermore, Cistanche increases the production of ATP itself, which is the molecule that gives energy to the whole organism; if ATP is missing, a whole series of subsystems, such as the immune system, do not function.

As regards DNA repair mechanisms, some of the substances in Cistanche appear to increase the repair rate, so more DNA is repaired faster; this is important because we know that DNA is constantly damaging itself all the time, every day, and more and more as time goes by.

It is also powerful as an immunostimulant, because it acts on different points of the immune system: at a cellular level, Cistanche polysaccharides enhance the phagocytic activity of macrophages.

One study showed that Cistanche significantly reduced the degree of mucosal hyperplasia and intestinal Helicobacter infections.

Cistanche has beneficial effects on bones in general because it decreases osteoclasts' activity and increases osteoblasts' activity.

A significant thing that Cistanche Deserticola does is reduce blood glucose levels, both fasting and after meals: this improves the effect of insulin resistance and dyslipidemia, which is known as a fatigue-fighting effect. Therefore, it reduces the accumulation of lactic acid and improves energy storage in the muscles.

When we talk about skin and hair, it turns out that Cistanche Deserticola can work wonders. It helps slow down the action of tyrosinase, collagenase, and elastase, which means our skin can stay more youthful and elastic as we age. Plus, when it comes to hair, several clinical studies show that people who take this supplement see a noticeable improvement in hair density and thickness after just four to five months.

The recommended daily dose for Cistanche extract is between 100 and 500 mg.

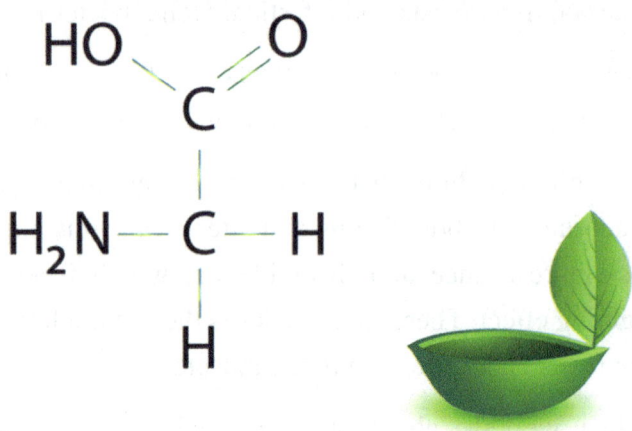

GLYCINE AND N-ACETYLCYSTEINE

Let's now talk about Glycine and N-acetylcysteine, a specific combination of two amino acids that has recently attracted attention for its ability to reverse several hallmarks of aging.

Glycine and N-acetylcysteine combined allow our body to produce its own antioxidants, promoting a more natural and balanced response to oxidative stress.

Dr. Premranjan Kumar, a pioneering researcher of Glycine and N-acetylcysteine studies, found that this unique combination of amino acids not only increases our internal production of antioxidants, but also rejuvenates the physical and cognitive functions of octogenarians to similar levels to those in their twenties.

We must first start with glutathione to understand the effect of Glycine and N-acetylcysteine combined. Glutathione is often referred to as the most powerful antioxidant, due to its unique properties and wide reach within the body.

Unlike other antioxidants targeting specific areas or functions, glutathione works systemically throughout the body, protecting cells, tissues, and organs. It also has the ability to regenerate other antioxidants, such as vitamins C and E, making it even more valuable in the fight against oxidative stress.

Glycine and N-acetylcysteine are two of the three precursors necessary to create the tripeptide glutathione; the third precursor is glutamate, which is abundant in most people, particularly in the central nervous system, and is involved in various aspects of normal brain function and cellular metabolism.

Glycine is an endogenous amino acid, meaning that the body can create it independently from other amino acids; it is a fundamental element for collagen, which makes up about a third of our skin, hair, bones, and joints. The average adult produces approximately 3 grams of Glycine daily, while the estimated daily requirement for optimal collagen synthesis is approximately 13 grams.

As we age, we lose up to 90 percent of collagen due to this Glycine deficiency and other factors such as genetics, environment, and lifestyle.

The other important substance for the creation of glutathione is N-acetylcysteine: it is a precursor of cysteine and is involved in numerous cellular processes; it protects cells from drugs and chemicals, and has been linked to a reduced risk of cancer, diabetes, respiratory problems, and infertility.

Since glutathione is considered the antioxidant par excellence, many people supplement glutathione directly; however, this may not be as effective as the integration of its precursors, Glycine and N-acetylcysteine.

The real advantage of these substances is that they support the cells in the production of their own glutathione: since different cells, in different organs, require different quantities of glutathione at different times, the integration of Glycine and N-acetylcysteine allows the cells to maintain their glutathione levels by producing as much as you need, when you need it.

It is very interesting to note that the supplementation of Glycine, or N-acetylcysteine, alone does not increase the production of glutathione, but the combination of the two does.

Who benefits most from supplementing with Glycine and N-acetylcysteine? Elderly people, people with chronic diseases, vegetarians and vegans.

DOSAGE: Glycine 500 mg and NAC 500 mg

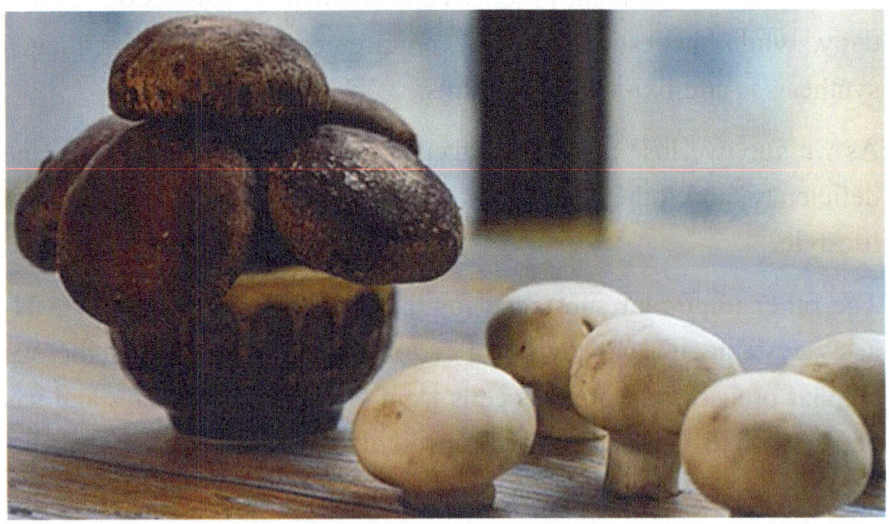

ERGOTHIONEINE

Ergothioneine is a natural amino acid derived from histidine with potent antioxidant properties. The human organism does not synthesize this amino acid independently, therefore it must integrate it.

Several studies have highlighted that ergothioneine:

- Can eliminate a wide range of reactive oxygen and nitrogen species;
- It has metal chelation properties; directly regulates the activity of nuclear factor erythroid 2-related factor 2 (Nrf2).

Ergothioneine not only enters the nucleus of our cells to protect our DNA, but it can also penetrate our mitochondria, the cell's powerhouses, where it acts as a potent intramitochondrial antioxidant—found in several foods like mushrooms, beans, oat bran, and fermented products, this compound is increasingly recognized as an important dietary nutrient for the prevention of a variety of inflammatory and cardiometabolic diseases.

Mushrooms are the richest source of ergothioneine, with varying amounts depending on the strain and growing conditions. Spirulina also contains relatively high quantities of this active ingredient.

You can also find supplements in powder or capsule form on the market.

DOSAGE: 5-20 mg per day

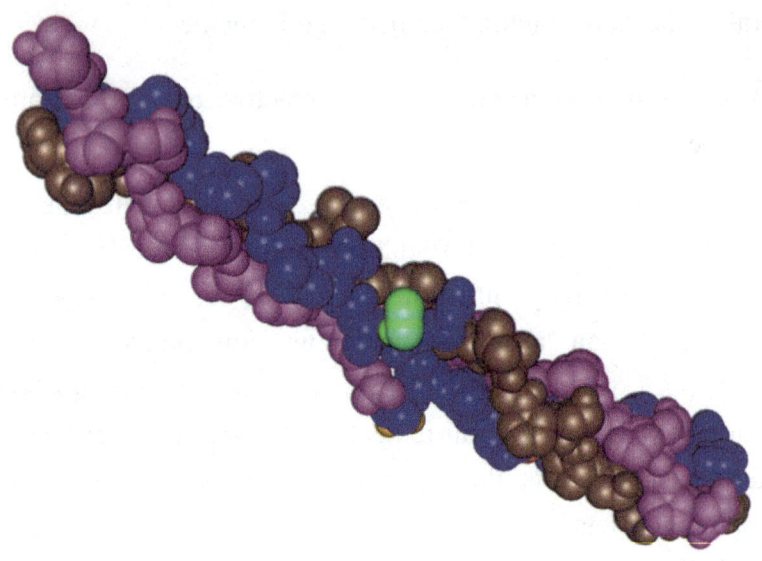

COLLAGEN

Collagen is a protein present throughout the human body. In particular, it is abundant in cartilage, bones, and, in general, in connective tissues. As time goes by, our body produces less and less collagen, and as a result, the skin loses firmness and elasticity.

For this reason, many think that taking collagen through supplements can slow down the skin's aging process. The problem is that, like all the proteins we take orally, our body dismantles the collagen protein into the various amino acids that compose it. Only a tiny part of these will actually be used to form new collagen. The cost/results ratio is, therefore, decidedly uninteresting.

Instead, taking those substances that induce the endogenous production of collagen, such as vitamin C, vitamin A, zinc, silicon, Omega3, and Quercetin, is more effective. In any case, it is essential that we consume sufficient proteins from our regular daily diet to ensure a sufficient supply of amino acids, and that we avoid sugar as much as possible, which is our skin's worst enemy.

If you really want to supplement, then prefer hydrolyzed collagen.

SUPPLEMENTATION PROGRAMS

Supplements (especially if they are quality ones) can cost a lot, so we propose some examples of supplement programs based on the importance of the supplement and the budget (assuming that you are already following an adequate diet and a correct lifestyle).

Low budget: Resveratrol (or Pterostilbene) Metformin (or Berberine) NAD Vit. D

Low-medium budget: Resveratrol (or Pterostilbene) Metformin (or Berberine) NAD Vit. D Omega 3 Magnesium Zinc

Medium budget: Resveratrol (or Pterostilbene) Metformin (or Berberine) NAD – Vit. D Omega 3 Magnesium Zinc Melatonin Folic acid

Medium-high budget: Resveratrol (or Pterostilbene) Metformin (or Berberine) NAD Vit. D Omega 3 Folic acid Magnesium – Zinc – Melatonin Astragalus Quercetin Curcumin Q10 Astaxanthin

In reality, supplementation should be personalized based on sex, age, weight, eating habits, lifestyle, etc.

For a custom program, write to fitnwellnesss@gmail.com

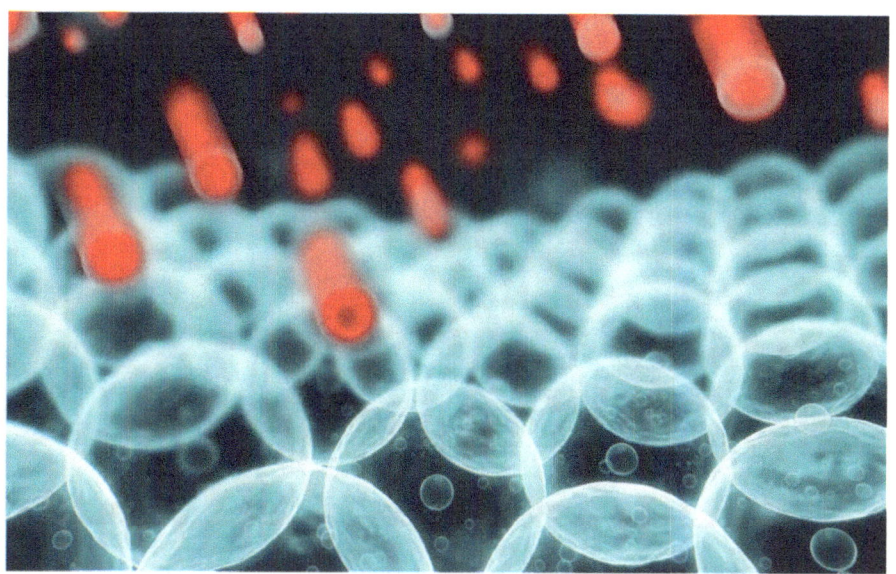

ANTI-FREE RADICALS

Fundamental substances to fight free radicals are alpha lipoic acid (the richest sources of alpha-lipoic acid are animal tissues with high metabolic activity such as red meat, heart, liver, and kidney among the vegetable sources there are, in decreasing way: spinach, broccoli, tomatoes, peas, Brussels sprouts, rice), glutathione (spinach, watermelon, grapefruit, and asparagus), pycnogenol (obtained from the bark of the French maritime pine), sulfur amino acids (such as cystine, cysteine, methionine), NAC (N-acetylcysteine), acetyl-L-carnitine, bioflavonoids, arginine, ornithine, OKG (ornithine alpha-ketoglutarate), glutamine, polyunsaturated fatty acids, beta-carotene, lutein, lycopene, zeaxanthin (carotenoids), resveratrol (in the coenzyme ubiquinol form).

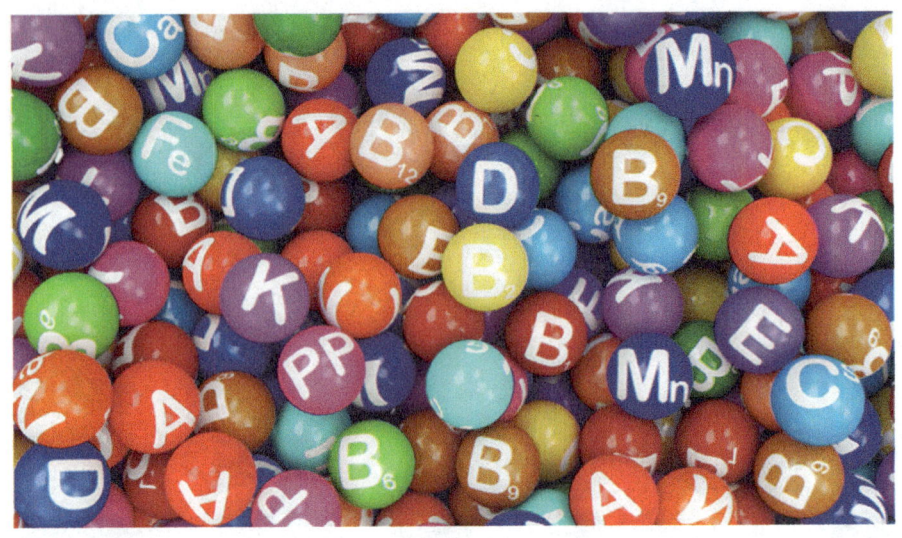

THE OTHER VITAMINS

There are several other vitamins that science is reevaluating, not just C, A, B, and E. Let's see the most important.

Vitamin I is present in brewer's yeast, cereals, and wheat germ; it regulates the cholesterol level and counteracts the alterations of the nervous system.

Vitamin U (or methyl methionine) is instead present in cabbage, asparagus, and celery, and is especially good for combating gastroesophageal reflux.

Instead, it has an anti-aging and antioxidant effect equal to that of the well-known vitamin E, the unknown vitamin T. It prevents vascular damage and is contained in a very high percentage in sesame, olive, hemp, and wheat germ oil.

Contained in vegetable fats such as soybean oil, hazelnuts, almonds, and avocados are vitamin M, which keeps cholesterol at bay.

And there is also vitamin O: it fights kidney and cardiovascular diseases, as well as Alzheimer's. Sources of vitamin O are red meat and dairy products, as well as seeds, legumes, artichokes, and broccoli.

Another important antioxidant is vitamin J or choline. It has a detoxifying and regenerating effect and is found in egg yolk, soy, and lettuce.

Finally, vitamin Z is actually a mineral contained in oysters, beans, pumpkin seeds, sunflower seeds, and mustard. It is considered the queen of vitamins because it helps the assimilation and absorption of all the others.

In any case, we always recommend that you consult your doctor before taking any supplement.

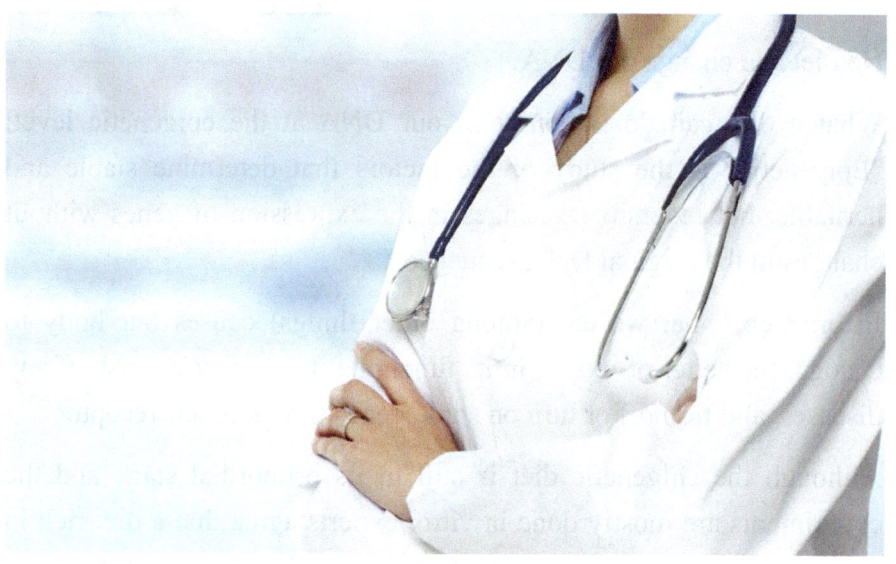

EPIGENETIC DIET

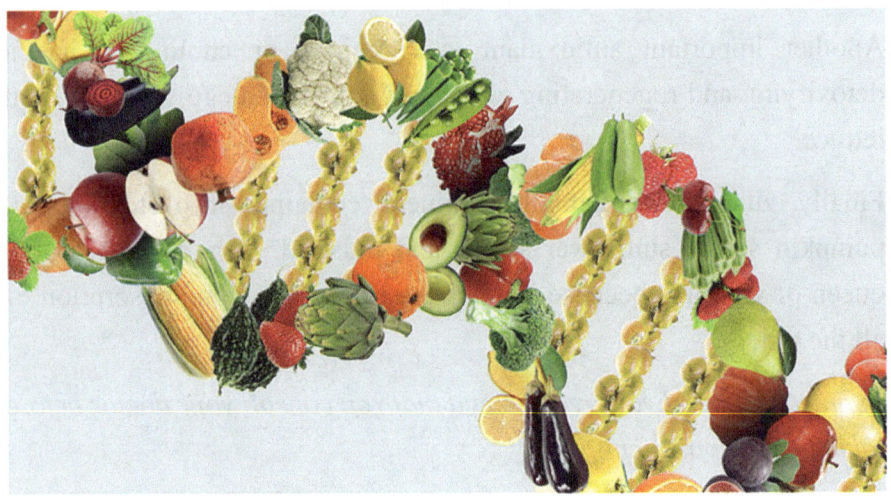

No diet can change our DNA.

What a diet can do is *condition* our DNA at the epigenetic level: "Epigenetics is the study of the factors that determine stable and heritable, but reversible, changes in the expression of genes without changes in the original DNA sequence."

In practice, what we eat (among other things) causes our body to change, for better or worse, in its functionality, correct the risk of any diseases, and turn off or turn on some genes through their receptors.

Although the epigenetic diet is still in its primordial stage and the experiments are mostly done in vitro, experts agree that a diet rich in particular substances such as cruciferous vegetables (cabbage, broccoli, arugula, chicory), soy, green tea, turmeric, vegetable fibers, could be useful to discourage the risk of certain diseases.

Although few things are known for sure about the epigenetic diet, it is good to know that the diet of our grandparents and fathers (indeed, to be precise, our grandmothers and our mothers) influenced our DNA, and that our diet and lifestyle will affect not only our health but also that of our children.

Formulating a "generic diet" is impossible, as diets must always be personalized for each individual.

In general, we can say that it is good to prefer those foods that counteract epigenetic drift. Among these substances, we find ECGC (which is the active substance of green tea), resveratrol, which is typical of red fruits and red wine, sulforaphane, which is the active substance of crucifers (therefore cabbage, broccoli, Brussels sprouts, etc.), and curcumin.

Recently, other naturally occurring substances in some foods, such as butyrate in certain goat cheeses, diallyl disulfide in garlic, and sulforaphane in broccoli, have been identified as inhibitors of Histone Deacetylase (HDAC).

Below is a non-exhaustive list of foods that should be included in an epigenetic diet:

CRUCIFEROUS VEGETABLES

They belong to the cruciferous family (whose correct botanical name is *Brassicaceae*): broccoli, cabbage of all kinds, turnip greens, horseradish, arugula, radishes, and watercress.

Among the benefits are the antibacterial, anti-inflammatory, and antioxidant properties, in addition to the high content of mineral salts, iron, calcium, and fiber.

In particular, broccoli is studied for its anti-cancer properties thanks to the high content of sulforaphane, which is a powerful anti-inflammatory.

In addition, broccoli is rich in vitamin C and vitamin K.

CELERY

Celery (*Apium graveolens*) is a herbaceous species belonging to the Apiaceae family. Celery is packed with nutrients and antioxidants, including vitamin C, vitamin A, potassium, folate, and flavonoids. It has anti-inflammatory, digestive, and satiating properties.

It reduces the risk of chronic diseases related to inflammation. Improve blood sugar and blood pressure levels.

PARSLEY

Parsley is a biennial plant of the *Apiaceae* family. It is very rich in vitamins, particularly C, A, K, folic acid, and other B vitamins, but it also boasts the presence of minerals, including potassium, calcium, and iron.

It has been seen how this aromatic herb acts positively on the functions of the liver, which helps in the purification of the organism.

It can then be helpful to keep blood sugar under control and, therefore, prevent the onset of type 2 diabetes, as well as regulate blood pressure.

Also rich in antioxidant substances, such as flavonoids, counteracts the action of free radicals and has an excellent anti-inflammatory effect. Parsley is also rich in beta-carotene (precursor of vitamin A), an antioxidant substance particularly beneficial for the health of the skin and eyes. If used raw, it is able to help digestion and reduce the production of intestinal gas; thanks to the presence of iron, it can counteract situations of slight anemia.

GREEN TEA

Green tea has a robust antioxidant action helpful in counteracting the action of free radicals, which are responsible for aging and diseases.

Green tea contains very high amounts of polyphenols, substances with a beneficial and antioxidant role for the human body; in particular, the most characteristic polyphenol and main responsible for the properties of green tea is epigallocatechin gallate (also known as EGCG, present in quantities about 10 times higher than black tea and 2.5 times higher than oolong tea).

Most of the benefits of green tea depend on the presence of large quantities of catechins, which are able to strengthen the antioxidant defenses and, therefore, reduce the damage to cells. In particular, it would have anti-tumor properties (protects good cells from mutations and inhibits the growth of cancerous ones) and would bring benefits to the cardiovascular system (inhibits the formation of clots, reduces the presence of fat and cholesterol in the blood, and slows the development of atherosclerosis and coronary heart disease) and respiratory.

Green tea also accelerates the metabolism of fats and sugars, facilitating the decrease in body weight and diuresis, and being useful in water retention, cellulite, and urinary tract infections.

Thanks to the combined action of polyphenolic derivatives (flavonoids, chlorogenic acid, caffeic acid, tannins) contained in it, this type of tea would have neuroprotective effects. It could play an important role in the prevention and treatment of neurodegenerative diseases.

Green tea also seems to be able to counteract hypertension and cause osteoporosis.

Green tea has plenty of health benefits, but it's important to remember that it contains caffeine. If you drink too much, it might cause anxiety, nervousness, and insomnia. Remember, green tea can also affect the functioning of the thyroid.

RED GRAPES

Grapes are a highly beneficial concentrate of flavonoids (natural antioxidants).

It has detoxifying properties, is antibacterial and anti-inflammatory, and strengthens the immune system.

The intake of grapes helps reduce bad cholesterol levels, counteracts constipation, strengthens capillaries, protects the venous walls, and is suitable for counteracting water retention and cellulite.

It contains resveratrol, a phenol found in the peel (which is why it is important to eat whole berries), and quercetin.

Thanks to the high content of boron, a substance that optimizes calcium absorption, it helps prevent osteoporosis.

Grapes can increase the level of leptin in the blood, the hormone that communicates a sense of satiety to the brain.

Levels of Vitamin C, K, and A are elevated.

SOY

Soy is a legume rich in proteins and polyunsaturated fats that are beneficial for health. It also provides essential minerals such as calcium, potassium, magnesium, iron, phosphorus, group A, B and C vitamins, and fiber.

Among the benefits that soy offers are intestinal regularity and the ability to keep blood sugar and cholesterol at bay. Thanks to the presence of mineral salts such as calcium and phosphorus, soy helps the mineralization of bones and prevents osteoporosis.

Thanks to the presence of isoflavones, it has proved useful in the female sphere for treating disorders related to menopause. Soy isoflavones compensate, at least partly, for the estrogens that tend to be lacking, creating imbalances in the female body when the woman is no longer fertile.

However, it has annoying contraindications if consumed in excess.

TOMATO

Tomatoes are a source of valuable nutrients, especially potassium, phosphorus, vitamin C, vitamin K, and folate. The red color of tomatoes is due to an antioxidant, lycopene (it is a carotenoid with an antioxidant action that is responsible for the red color of tomatoes and other vegetables such as watermelon and red fruits it has anti-inflammatory activity and protects the eyes from degeneration due to age its strong antioxidant power makes it valuable in the fight against both cellular aging and cancer lycopene is mainly contained in the peel), whose action is assisted by two other antioxidants: lutein and zeaxanthin (these are two carotenoids that are present inside the retina where, thanks to their antioxidant action, they protect the eyes from radiation damage).

BEANS

Beans are the fruits of a plant of the legume family, *Phaseolus vulgaris L.*, native to Central America.

Numerous cultivated varieties are known, and all contain *phytohemagglutinin*, a toxic protein destroyed during cooking.

Beans are very nutritious and rich in vitamins A, B, C, and E; they also contain mineral and trace mineral salts, such as potassium, iron, calcium, zinc, and phosphorus. Since beans are legumes, they are rich in lecithin, a phospholipid that promotes the emulsion of fats, avoiding their accumulation in the blood and consequently reducing the level of cholesterol.

All types of beans contain a lot of fiber, but some varieties have plenty: black beans, for example, contain 6 grams of fiber per half-cup serving, common beans are around 7 grams, and with cowpea beans, it comes to 8 grams.

Canned beans are as good as dry beans but are high in sodium, so drain and rinse them before consuming. Fiber is precious for metabolism and helps to reach the feeling of satiety easily. Beans are made up of 60% starches and sugars, while green beans are made up of 90% water; therefore, their protein content is significantly lower than that of beans; however, they contain a greater amount of mineral salts and vitamin A.

CAPERS

Capers are the buds of *Capparis spinosa*, a species native to the Mediterranean region belonging to the Capparaceae family.

Capers are a source of antioxidants: quercetin is endowed with antibacterial, anticancer, analgesic, and anti-inflammatory properties, while rutin strengthens capillaries and inhibits the formation of platelet aggregates, thus promoting good circulation in the smallest blood vessels.

They contain vitamin A, vitamin C, vitamin E, niacin, riboflavin, vitamin B6, thiamine, pantothenic acid, vitamin K, folate, sodium, potassium, calcium, magnesium, phosphorus, iron, copper, zinc, manganese, selenium.

SPINACH

The spinach we eat is the edible leaves of the herbaceous plant *Spinacia oleracea*.

Spinach is rich in vitamin A and folic acid. They are also rich in nitrate, a substance that is the subject of recent research as it appears to increase the energy level available in the body. They also contain lutein, which is helpful for the retina's and eyes' health.

Spinach contains iron, but the belief that it brings a high amount of it to the body is wrong. It is advisable to consume spinach seasoned with lemon to facilitate the absorption of this mineral; in fact, the vitamin C contained in citrus helps to absorb iron.

On the contrary, potassium is abundant.

Among other compounds, oxalic acid and antioxidants such as beta-carotene, lutein, zeaxanthin, and quercetin should be noted.

They are also precious for the presence of an amino acid, tyrosine, which acts on the brain by promoting the production of dopamine and norepinephrine, two important neurotransmitters.

ARUGULA

Arugula is an herbaceous plant belonging to the Cruciferae family. It is rich in micronutrients, such as calcium, potassium, folate, and vitamins K, A and C. It has a powerful antioxidant and anti-inflammatory activity. It is low in calories and high in fiber.

This vibrant green has numerous valuable nutrients for the health and functioning of bones, heart, eyes, and immune system. Plus, it reduces oxidative stress and the inflammatory state and lowers the risk of cardiovascular, cancer, and aging-related diseases.

Arugula also aids digestion (the bitter substances of which it is composed stimulate the production of gastric juices, facilitating digestion), and finally, it has relaxing properties and helps promote sleep.

WALNUTS

Walnuts are the fruit of the trees of the genus *Juglans*.

Walnut is properly a tonic nervous system and possesses anti-anemic, antispasmodic, sedative, and anti-inflammatory properties. The cardiac effect of walnuts depends on the balance in electrolytes and, above all, on their action on the elastic tone of the vessels that favor arterial circulation.

They are a source of Omega 3, fiber, antioxidants including vitamin E, and mineral salts such as magnesium.

They are rich in mineral salts such as iron, calcium, magnesium, potassium, fluorine, copper, zinc, and phosphorus. They have a high content of unsaturated fats, or "good fats," including oleic acid, Omega 3, and Omega 6, which are especially important for reducing cholesterol. They contain valuable antioxidants such as tocopherols (vitamin E), polyphenols, tannins, and flavonoids. They provide inulin with a beneficial effect on digestion. They provide melatonin and tryptophan, an amino acid necessary for the production of serotonin, which is good for the health of the nervous system.

Habitual consumption of walnuts can also have a protective effect against neurodegenerative diseases and lead to an improvement in cognitive functions, especially in the elderly population.

The effect would be due to the high content of unsaturated fats and antioxidants, which are able to reduce inflammatory and oxidative processes in the cells of the nervous system and block the development of degenerative ones in neurons.

GARLIC

Garlic (*Allium sativum L*) belongs to the Liliaceae family.

A garlic clove is a reservoir of highly effective healing active ingredients such as allicin, sulfur, and B vitamins. It has anti-helminthic properties against roundworms and pinworms, anti-mucolytic, hypotensive, expectorant, digestive, carminative, antiseptic, and hypoglycemic.

The role of this plant in regulating cholesterol and triglycerides and improving the relationship between LDL cholesterol and HDL cholesterol has now been widely demonstrated.

Allicin (sulfur compound contained in garlic) is a remarkable antibiotic whose strong inhibitory power on numerous types of bacteria was noted by Louis Pasteur as early as 1858.

In addition to allicin, garlic contains other antibacterial substances such as garlicina; it is rich in minerals, such as magnesium, calcium, phosphorus, iodine, and iron; there are traces of zinc, manganese, selenium, vitamin C (only in fresh garlic), provitamin A, vitamins B1-B2-PP; contains hormone-like substances and enzymes (lysozyme and peroxidase).

Garlic also contains alkaloids that perform an action similar to insulin, lowering the blood sugar level.

SAUERKRAUT

Sauerkraut is a typical side dish of German cuisine, obtained from cabbage, finely chopped, and subjected to lactic fermentation.

Rich in vitamins, mineral salts, and amino acids, sauerkraut is a powerful ally of intestinal well-being as it promotes digestion and strengthens intestinal flora. Thanks to the lactic acid contained, sauerkraut is a kind of natural probiotic.

Another aspect that makes sauerkraut special is the high content of vitamin K, and the essential vitamin C. Sauerkraut is also rich in folic acid-vitamin B9, which stimulates the use of this vitamin in the body.

They are also rich in choline (vitamin J), a substance potentially helpful in reducing circulating homocysteine as a cardiovascular risk factor. Sauerkraut, using bacterial fermentation, also contains good quantities of cobalamin (vitamin B12), a limiting factor in strict vegan diets.

SALMON

Salmon is an excellent source of protein, vitamins (vitamin B6, vitamin B12, thiamin, niacin), minerals (phosphorus, selenium), and omega-3 fatty acids.

Phosphorus is essential for the health of bones and teeth, while selenium allows cellular antioxidants to function correctly.

Vitamin B6 stimulates brain functions and prevents aging; vitamin B12 plays a valuable role in producing red blood cells and forming the bone marrow. Niacin (or vitamin B3) promotes circulation, protects the skin, and promotes the digestion of food. Thiamine (or vitamin B1) releases a good body energy source.

Omega 3s (fatty acids in which this fish is very rich) reduce the risk of heart attack, and cardiovascular and coronary diseases, thin the blood, lower the risk of stroke, and have an antiarrhythmic effect on the heart. In the case of prolonged intake, they reduce triglycerides and, over the years, the risk of thrombosis.

DHA is a very important fatty acid, an essential component of the retina (it constitutes about 50%): its role is fundamental in the well-being of sight. Eating salmon, which is the richest fish in DHA, is therefore good for the eyes. In particular, it has been observed that feeding at least 2-3 times a week with this food slows down the degeneration of a specific area of the retina, the macula lutea, which is often observed with the passing of the years.

Eating salmon improves sleep. This type of fish, in fact, contains tryptophan, a substance that has a sedating effect and can help, in particular, to fight insomnia and fall asleep faster.

A valid contribution is also given by vitamin B6, which is rich in salmon and capable of promoting melatonin production.

APPLES

Apple contains no fat or protein, very few calories, and even less sugar.

On the other hand, it is rich in mineral salts and B vitamins, so it is good for the intestinal mucous membranes, prevents the impoverishment of nails and hair, and fights fatigue. In addition, the apple fibers help the body protect itself against external attacks. Citric and malic acids also contribute to the well-being of the person, particularly the digestive system, because they facilitate digestion and keep acidity unchanged.

Apples are rich in polyphenols, which counteract the action of free radicals in the body, the cause of cellular aging; in addition, they also have the advantage of lowering the cholesterol content in the blood thanks to pectin, thus saving the cardiovascular system in general.

The beneficial action of apples also extends to the field of cancer prevention, thanks to the flavonoid content and vitamin C.

Apple can not only reduce the absorption of "bad" cholesterol, as has been shown in numerous studies, but also lower blood glucose levels. Finally, it slows down oxidative stress and premature cell aging, thanks to quercetins and proanthocyanidins.

NB: apples must be eaten with the peel, since most of the insoluble fiber and many of the typical antioxidants of the apple are present in the peel.

AVOCADO

From a botanical point of view, the avocado fruit is a drupe, like peach, apricot, cherry, olive, and coconut.

Avocado is rich in monounsaturated fatty acids (MUFA), antioxidants, and fiber. It features a good amount of vitamins and minerals, including vitamin A, vitamin C, vitamin E, iron, potassium, calcium, and magnesium.

It reduces LDL (bad) cholesterol levels, favoring the increase of HDL (good) cholesterol. It reduces the risk of developing Metabolic Syndrome, a disease characterized by the coexistence of several factors, including hyperglycemia, dyslipidemia, and hypertension.

It promotes intestinal transit and improves blood sugar and fat levels.

It reduces inflammation and, therefore, the risk of developing associated diseases.

Avocados are fiber-rich, which, unlike oils, contributes to satiety. It also helps the body absorb fat-soluble vitamins introduced with meals, such as A, E, and K.

Compared to other tropical fruits such as coconut and oil palm, the percentage of saturated fat in avocado is more modest.

Instead, the monounsaturated component prevails, with a strong presence of Omega 9 oleic acid, the same fat that characterizes extra virgin olive oil and to which many metabolic benefits are attributed.

BLUEBERRIES

Several properties are attributed to the blueberry, such as astringent, antioxidant, vasoprotective, lipid-lowering, hypoglycemic, antiseptic, and antiviral properties.

Bilberry has also been shown to exert protective action at the endothelium of arterial vessels and capillaries from damage caused by diabetes and hypertension. More specifically, this activity is carried out by the anthocyanosides contained in the blueberry fruits.

Anthocyanosides also reduce platelet aggregation induced by ADP, collagen, PAF, and arachidonic acid; they have vigorous antioxidant activity; they protect the gastric mucosa from inflammatory or irritative stimuli, and have beneficial effects on sight.

The berries of the bilberry contain many organic acids (malic, citric, etc.), tannins, pectin, vitamins A and C, and, to a lesser extent, vitamin B and anthocyanin glycosides (*mirtillin*), which reduce the permeability of capillaries and strengthen the structure of connective tissue, which supports blood vessels, improving their elasticity and tone.

These principles contained in the phytocomplex give it the capillary protective property, making it particularly suitable for treating circulatory disorders, especially of venous origin, and in all cases of capillary fragility, primarily affecting the retina.

Anthocyanins can inhibit the activity of some enzymes that destroy collagen and the elastic tissues of the capillaries and vessels of the peripheral circulatory system, causing fragility and excessive permeability.

The vast nutritional qualities of blueberry also derive from the rich presence of vitamins A, C, B1, B2, PP, and essential mineral salts for our body (calcium, phosphorus, iron, sodium, and potassium).

In addition to being an excellent source of vitamin C, this fruit is among the best natural sources of antioxidants and appears to have protective properties for the bladder and urinary tract (in particular, it reduces the risk of bacterial infections), and it seems to promote normal digestive function.

GOAT MILK

Goat's milk globules are smaller and have a larger surface area, making them more attackable by intestinal lipases, improving lipid metabolism, and reducing the level of triglycerides.

It has low levels of casein, as in human milk, and high taurine levels. It promotes the bile secretion of cholesterol.

It has a high quantity of short and medium-chain fatty acids, such as butyric acid, and has an anticancer action.

It has a high L-carnitine content, resulting in better utilization of fats at the mitochondrial level.

High content of calcium, phosphorus, selenium, and zinc, as well.

MUSHROOMS

Mushrooms are biologically distinct from foods of plant and animal origin, with a unique nutritional profile.

Their consumption is growing among those who choose an epigenetic diet, given the ability to reduce the intake of calories, saturated fatty acids, and sodium and increase the intake of nutrients such as fiber, potassium, and vitamin D.

In particular, they are rich in copper, phosphorus, potassium, selenium, zinc, riboflavin, niacin, choline, iron, thiamine, folate, and vitamin B6.

Few foods naturally contain vitamin D, and mushrooms are unique in this.

A portion of raw mushrooms, exposed to UV rays, can contain 23.6 µg to 25.52 µg of vitamin D. Mushrooms are also one of the best food sources of two antioxidants: the sulfur amino acid ergothioneine and glutathione.

TYPICALLY ANTIOXIDANT FOODS

Nutraceuticals, the science that studies the medicinal properties of foods, indicates that most of the antioxidants are found in plant products; these are mainly polyphenols (such as catechin, isoflavones, resveratrol), carotenoids (such as lycopene and lutein), vitamins (A, C, and E).

Then oranges, carrots, black and red grapes (the peel contains resveratrol), dog rose, tomato (do not clean the gelatinous part and the seeds), pineapple, lemon, green salads, sprouts, wheat germ, nettle, pomegranate (even richer antioxidants and resveratrol from wine), parsley, fennel, cucumber, melon, pumpkin, spinach, broccoli, papaya, apricot, blueberry, strawberry, grapefruit, cauliflower, green tea.

Other anti-aging foods are artichokes (rich in inulin, luteinam polyphenols; they also have purifying effects, probiotics beneficial for the intestinal flora), beans (in addition to being rich in vegetable proteins, they have a good antioxidant power, in particular red and black beans, also with an excellent content of useful minerals), lentils, soy, chickpeas, peas, garlic (the anti-aging power is mainly due to allicin, an antibiotic and antifungal substance, also with anti-cholesterol properties), plums (high presence of vitamin C and E, beta-carotene, polyphenols and flavonols), dried fruit (vitamin E, folate, polyunsaturated fatty acids such as Omega 3: walnuts, hazelnuts, almonds, pistachios, pecans), apples (rich in flavonoids such as quercetin, epicatechin and procyanidin), cocoa (many polyphenols and flavonoids in particular epicatechin; polyphenols play a key role in keeping the brain young), tea (the catechins present in tea help fight oxidative stress), avocado (very rich in vitamins A and E, antioxidants; also it is a good source of Omega 3), sultanas and other dehydrated fruits such as plums, dates and figs, are a concentrate of antioxidants, much richer in polyphenols and vitamins C and E than fresh counterparts, asparagus (known for their purifying and diuretic properties are also helpful in fighting free radicals thanks to the presence of vitamin A, C and glutathione asparagus has more flavonoids than broccoli unfortunately boiling asparagus for a long time significantly decreases their antioxidant value, therefore you must avoid overcooking them), whole grains (they provide fiber and antioxidants; rich in phenolic acids, flavonoids, vitamin E and B vitamins you can choose from the many varieties of rice, barley, spelled, oats, rye, quinoa and buckwheat).

We remind you that before embarking on a diet and/or taking any supplement, you must seek your doctor's advice or a specialist.

As well as it is always helpful to carry out specific blood tests to assess any deficiencies or problems.

Another useful test is the **mineralogram**, which evaluates the toxic minerals and metals deposited in the body. It is a test that measures the mineral content in the hair and, consequently, in the body tissues.

After carrying out the examination, if deficiencies are found, supplementation is followed for 4-6 months, then the test is repeated.

In the case of excess heavy metals, such as aluminum, mercury, lead, and cadmium, the only way to remove them is *chelation therapy.*

This is the most potent antioxidant therapy and uses the intravenous use of E.D.T.A. (ethyl diamino tetraacetic acid) and other antioxidants.

The book "Complementary Therapies Antiaging" lists alternative and natural techniques for longevity.

In the book "Antiaging Recipes," you will find some easy and tasty recipes for an epigenetic diet.

COSMETICS

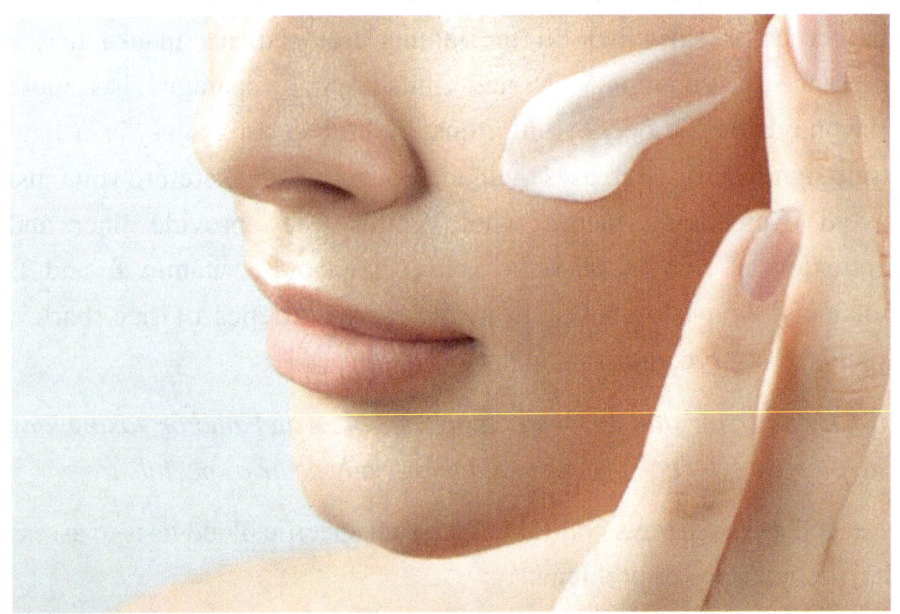

Modern cosmetic science nowadays puts safe and highly effective products at our disposal to reduce the appearance of wrinkles, counteract the loss of hydration, tone, and elasticity, and fight the free radicals responsible for a large part of skin aging.

Let us then see what the ingredients of the truly effective anti-aging cosmetic products available on the market are.

HYALURONIC ACID

Hyaluronic acid plays a fundamental role in anti-aging preparations, whether for topical or nutricosmetics use.

According to what is reported in scientific literature, topical formulations based on hyaluronic acid (creams, gels, lotions, serums, fillers, etc.) show good effectiveness, especially in terms of hydrating, firming and re-densifying action on mature skin: hyaluronic acid, in fact, it not only helps to retain water at the skin level, thus keeping it hydrated, but also stimulates the synthesis of collagen and elastin, thus contributing to the maintenance of tone and elasticity. Hyaluronic acid can be used without the risk of developing allergic reactions (except for individual hypersensitivities) since it is a molecule naturally present in the extracellular matrix: for this reason, it is also widely used in cosmetic surgery. Nevertheless, be careful: non-allergenicity applies to hyaluronic acid itself, not to other additives that may be present in the final product, which allergy sufferers must always pay attention to.

Within cosmetic formulations, hyaluronic acid is used in concentrations between 0.2 and 1%, alone or in association with other active ingredients with synergistic action (vitamins, peptides, probiotics, plant extracts).

PEPTIDES

Peptides are short chains of amino acids that form the building blocks of proteins like collagen, elastin, and keratin, all of which are essential for keeping skin firm, elastic, and youthful. As we age, the production of these proteins decreases, leading to wrinkles, sagging, and loss of tone. Applying peptides can help stimulate collagen production and improve skin structure.

Peptides act in various ways depending on the type. They can:

1. Stimulate collagen production: Some peptides send signals to skin cells to increase collagen production, improving skin structure and reducing wrinkles.

2. Strengthen the skin barrier: Peptides help maintain a healthy skin barrier, preventing moisture loss and protecting the skin from harmful external agents.

3. Reduce inflammation: Certain peptides have anti-inflammatory properties, which can soothe the skin and improve its resilience to environmental stress.

4. Increase elasticity: Specific peptides can enhance skin elasticity, making it firmer and reducing sagging.

There are different types of peptides used in skincare products and aesthetic medicine. Here are the main ones:

1. Signal peptides: These peptides send signals to skin cells to boost collagen and other structural components. One of the most well-known is palmitoyl pentapeptide-4 (Matrixyl), commonly used in anti-aging serums.

2. Carrier peptides: Carrier peptides transport essential minerals like copper and magnesium into skin cells, stimulating collagen production and improving repair. A common example is copper peptide (GHK-Cu), which has powerful regenerative and antioxidant effects.

3. Enzyme-inhibitor peptides: These peptides help block enzymes that break down collagen, such as matrix metalloproteinases, preserving skin structure.

4. Neurotransmitter peptides (botox-like): These peptides reduce facial muscle contractions, minimizing the appearance of expression lines. The most famous is acetyl hexapeptide-8 (Argireline), known as a less invasive alternative to botox.

Benefits of peptides for the skin:

Wrinkle reduction: By stimulating collagen and elastin production, peptides can improve skin structure and reduce the appearance of fine lines and wrinkles.

Improved elasticity: More elastic skin means less sagging and a more youthful, toned appearance.

Hydration and barrier reinforcement: Strengthening the skin's protective barrier helps prevent moisture loss and improves the overall look of the skin.

Antioxidant effects: Some peptides, like GHK-Cu, have powerful antioxidant effects that protect the skin from free radical damage.

Peptides can be combined with other anti-aging ingredients to maximize results, such as:

Retinol: Further stimulates collagen production.

Hyaluronic acid: Improves hydration and skin firmness.

Vitamin C: A powerful antioxidant that boosts collagen and brightens the skin.

NB: choose formulations that contain a diversified pool of peptides and at a concentration of no less than 3%.

VITAMINS AND ANTIOXIDANTS

Vitamins C, A, E, group B, polyphenols, resveratrol, caffeic acid, and Coenzyme Q are all ingredients with an antioxidant action that we can find in anti-aging formulations.

We know that among those responsible for skin aging, free radicals play a prominent role in the oxidative stress they generate, counteracting their harmful effects, which, therefore, can translate into effective action against the skin blemishes caused by them.

Vitamin C (ascorbic acid) and vitamin E (tocopherol) are among the most powerful antioxidants that we host within our body; furthermore, vitamin C is essential for collagen synthesis, the actual "scaffold" of our skin. It stimulates the action of microcirculation, which in turn guarantees the constant supply of oxygen and nutrients to the skin and the correct disposal of waste substances.

Vitamin A (retinol) and retinoids (its derivatives, natural or synthetic), in addition to their antioxidant action, stimulate collagen production and reduce damage from exposure to UV rays.

Vitamin B3 (nicotinamide or niacinamide) contributes to the repair of damage from UVA and UVB radiation; in some clinical trials, the daily application of a cream containing 5% niacinamide produced, after 12 weeks, a significant improvement in terms of increased skin elasticity and reduction of wrinkles.

Coenzyme Q10 is an essential co-factor in numerous enzymatic ratios within the cells of the human body; in addition to this, it is a good antioxidant and stimulant of collagen synthesis and, applied topically, also seems to have a role in the reduction of wrinkles.

SUBSTANCES WITH A HYDRATING ACTION

In addition to the aforementioned hyaluronic acid, there are numerous oils and fats of mineral or vegetable origin capable of replenishing and maintaining the good conditions of the hydrolipidic film, the natural emulsion that covers our skin and which protects it from external agents and excessive dehydration: among the former, we remember paraffin (vaseline), among the latter:

- argan oil
- olive oil
- castor oil
- shea butter

Glycerin also has an effective hydrating action, as does panthenol (pro-vitamin B5).

FOSPIDINA.

Fospidina is the latest generation active complex that boasts a scientific study resulting from over 30 years of research in cell biology and dermatology. It is made up of phospholipids extracted from soy and glucosamine. This is so effective because glucosamine, a precursor of hyaluronic acid, is carried by phospholipids that penetrate the deeper layers of the dermis.

Compared to creams with hyaluronic acid, creams with Fospidina offer the advantage of a smaller molecule supported by efficient "carriers" such as phospholipids, which is why glucosamine penetrates better through the epidermis to develop all its regenerating action deeply. The result is a complex that acts both as an anti-aging active ingredient and as a carrier to maximize the performance of the other ingredients.

Its active ingredients are divided into:

Phospholipids

- Fundamental constituents of cell membranes.
- High conveying power with carrier action.
- Rich in linoleic and linolenic acid, it is useful for the integrity of the surface hydrolipidic barrier.
- They promote cell regeneration.

Glucosamine

- Participates in the constitution of cell membranes.
- Precursor of hyaluronic acid.

In any case, the essential and most crucial face and body cream to use to slow down the aging of our skin is undoubtedly the sun cream (of proven quality) with a high protection anti-UV filter (even in winter!).

Although there are many causes of skin aging, the damage caused by sun exposure is largely the most harmful.

CONCLUSIONS

In summary, the fundamental pillars for achieving a *healthy life for as long as possible* are:

- Regular physical activity
- Nutrition The key is to eat healthy foods (with low glycemic impact) and eat little (slightly below your TDEE) (Contributors to Wikimedia projects, 2023)
- Quality sleep
- No alcohol No smoking
- Stress management
- Social relationships and care for your mental/emotional well-being
- Supplementation
- Low inflammation

But let's remember that the issue does not have the "right diet"; the issue is "doing the diet."

The issue is not having proof of how much smoking, drinking alcohol, or consuming sugar is bad for us; the issue is stopping doing it.

And stopping forever!

The issue is not having all the information possible; the issue is putting the information acquired into practice.

In the end, it all boils down to a neuro-psychological problem, that is, the problem of "change."

Without motivation, action, determination, and perseverance, no change is achieved.

DISCLAIMER

The content of this book has been checked and compiled with the utmost care. The contents' completeness, correctness, and topicality have been considered throughout the making of this book; however, it is impossible to guarantee the success of actions based on the book's contents. The content of this book is a synthesis of decades of scientific research, but it should be distinct from medical help. There will be no legal liability or liability for damages resulting from counterproductive exercises or errors on the reader's part. No guarantee can be given for success. The author, therefore, assumes no responsibility for the failure to achieve the objectives described in the book.

Sources: Life Extension Movement – PubMed – Dr. Carlotta Gnavi – My Personal Trainer – Natural cures – INNsite – Near future – Magazine X115 – Healthspring – Humanitas – Farmastar – Dcomedieta – Esquire – Anagen – Medical News – The Wom Healthy – Skinius – Wim Hof – Valerio Rosso – Dr. Peter Attia

© 2024

REFERENCES

Contributors to Wikimedia projects. (2001, August 15). Eukaryote Wikipedia. Wikipedia, the free encyclopedia. https://en.wikipedia.org/wiki/Eukaryote

Contributors to Wikimedia projects. (2003, October 6). Cortisol Wikipedia. Wikipedia, the free encyclopedia. https://en.wikipedia.org/wiki/Cortisol

Contributors to Wikimedia projects. (2002, February 25). Histone Wikipedia. Wikipedia, the free encyclopedia. https://en.wikipedia.org/wiki/Histone

Contributors to Wikimedia projects. (2005, January 19). High-intensity interval training Wikipedia. Wikipedia, the free encyclopedia. https://en.wikipedia.org/wiki/High-intensity_interval_training

Contributors to Wikimedia projects. (2023, October 15). Energy expenditure Wikipedia. Wikipedia, the free encyclopedia. https://en.wikipedia.org/wiki/Energy_expenditure

Homocysteine Test: MedlinePlus Medical Test. (n.d.). MedlinePlus Health Information from the National Library of Medicine. https://medlineplus.gov/lab-tests/homocysteine-test/

Johnson, J. (2020, May 27). What is diaphragmatic breathing? Benefits and how-to. Medical and health information | MedicalNewsToday. https://www.medicalnewstoday.com/articles/diaphragmatic-breathing#conditions-it-can-help-with

ScienceDirect. (n.d.). Insulin sensitivity. In Topics in medicine and dentistry. Retrieved October 11, 2024, from https://www.sciencedirect.com/topics/medicine-and-dentistry/insulin-sensitivity

VO2 Max Testing Exercise Physiology Core Laboratory. (n.d.). Exercise Physiology Core Laboratory. https://med.virginia.edu/exercise-physiology-core-laboratory/fitness-assessment-for-community-members/vo2-max-testing/

Made in the USA
Monee, IL
01 December 2024

71787571R20066